D0718831

**Norris and
Campbell's
Nurse's Guide to
Anaesthetics,
Resuscitation and
Intensive Care**

CHURCHILL LIVINGSTONE NURSING TEXTS

Nutrition and Dietetics for Nurses
Sixth edition
Mary E. Beck

Principles of Infection and Immunity in Patient Care
Caroline Blackwell and D. M. Weir

Practical Therapeutics for Nursing and Related Professions
Third edition
James A. Boyle

Practical Notes on Nursing Procedures
Seventh edition
J. D. Britten

Bacteriology and Immunity for Nurses
Fifth edition
Ronald Hare and E. Mary Cooke

Drugs and Pharmacology for Nurses
Seventh edition
S. J. Hopkins

Essentials of Paediatrics for Nurses
Fifth edition
I. Kessel

Psychology as Applied to Nursing
Seventh edition
Andrew McGhie

Anatomy and Physiology Applied to Nursing
Fifth edition
Janet T. E. Riddle

Principles of Nursing
Second edition
Nancy Roper

Foundations of Nursing and First Aid
Fifth edition
Janet S. Ross and Kathleen J. W. Wilson

Norris and Campbell's Nurse's Guide to Anaesthetics, Resuscitation and Intensive Care

Donald Campbell

M.B.Ch.B., F.F.A.R.C.S., D.A., F.R.C.P. (Glas.)
Professor of Anaesthesia, University of Glasgow
Honorary Consultant Anaesthetist, Glasgow
Royal Infirmary

Alastair A. Spence

M.D., F.F.A.R.C.S., M.R.C.P. (Glas.)
Professor, University of Glasgow
Honorary Consultant Anaesthetist, Western Infirmary, Glasgow

SEVENTH EDITION

Churchill Livingstone 🏛

EDINBURGH LONDON MELBOURNE AND NEW YORK 1983

CHURCHILL LIVINGSTONE
Medical Division of Longman Group Limited

Distributed in the United States of America by
Churchill Livingstone Inc., 1560 Broadway, New York,
N.Y. 10036, and by associated companies,
branches and representatives throughout
the world.

First edition 1964   Fifth edition 1972
Second edition 1965   Sixth edition 1975
Third edition 1967   Seventh edition 1983
Fourth edition 1969

ISBN 0 443 02721 8

British Library Cataloguing in Publication Data
Norris, Walter
    Norris and Campbell's nurse's guide to
    anaesthetics, resuscitation and intensive care.
    — 7th ed. — (Churchill Livingstone nursing
    texts)
1. Anaesthesia
I. Title II. Campbell, Donald, 1930–
III. Spence, Alastair A.
    617'.96'024613   RD81

Library of Congress Cataloging in Publication Data
Norris, Walter.
    Norris and Campbell's Nurse's guide to
anaesthetics, resuscitation, and intensive
care.
    (Churchill Livingstone nursing texts)
    Includes index.
    1. Anaesthesia. 2. Surgical nursing.
3. Resuscitation. 4. Intensive care nursing. I. Campbell, Donald, 1930– . II. Spence,
Alastair A. III. Title. IV. Title: Nurse's guide to anaesthetics, resuscitation, and intensive
care. V. Series. [DNLM: 1. Anaesthesiology—Nursing texts. 2. Intensive care
units—Nursing texts. 3. Nursing care. 4. Resuscitation—Nursing texts. WY 151
N854n] RD82.N66 1982 617'.96'024613 82-1267
                                        AACR2

Printed in Singapore by
Selector Printing Co Pte Ltd.

Preface to the Seventh Edition

The continuing usefulness of a book such as this, developed to assist those involved in the rapidly changing scene in anaesthesia and intensive care, must inevitably depend on frequent and often quite substantial revision. This must be achieved without losing sight of the original aims as outlined in the Preface to the First Edition so many years ago. The present edition has accordingly been extensively revised and new illustrative material included. As before the authors have benefited from the constructive criticism of colleagues both nursing and medical and would wish again to express their appreciation of this continuing interest. The new format of the book on this occasion will, we hope, aid reference to selected topics in the text and the authors are indebted to the publishers for their advice and help in this respect. We also wish to thank our secretaries Miss E. Polly and Mrs Janette Buttar for their help in the preparation of the manuscript.

Glasgow, 1983

D.C.
A.A.S.

Preface to the First Edition

In this country nurses are not called upon to administer anaesthetics but the part they play in the care of the patient before, during and after anaesthesia is nevertheless an important one. We have tried to set out in this book some of the methods used by the present day anaesthetist, explaining how these affect the nursing care of the patient.

The routine pre-anaesthetic preparation and supervision of the patient is discussed and illustrated and it is hoped that in this way the nurse will understand and remember easily the reasons that lie behind the various methods.

The increasing use of recovery rooms and intensive care units has called for the training of nurses in the special techniques used in such units and a description of some of the methods is included.

Finally, it is considered appropriate to include in this work a description of the techniques of resuscitation currently taught, as it is often the nurse who has the first, and indeed sometimes the only opportunity to apply these successfully. Neither lectures nor text-books can replace practical demonstrations of anaesthetic apparatus and its maintenance nor the essentially practical techniques of resuscitation. These must be learned 'in the field'.

While minor variations of technique may exist from hospital to hospital there is no disagreement on the fundamental principles which we have tried to present to our readers.

This book is based on lectures delivered by the authors at the Glasgow Royal Infirmary and Associated Hospitals, Gartloch Hospital, and the Royal College of Nursing, Edinburgh.

1964   W. Norris
                                                                  D. Campbell

Contents

1

Historical introduction

Nowadays, the patient entering hospital to undergo surgical treatment can be assured that there will be no pain during the operation. This was not always so; until the middle of the nineteenth century anyone unfortunate enough to require an operation was fortified beforehand by alcohol in some form and was held down by strong men during the actual surgical procedure. Mercifully the pain was often so severe that the patient fainted and to this extent was spared some of the agony. It is not surprising therefore that such operations as were performed were restricted to life-saving procedures that could be undertaken very rapidly. A common example was the amputation of a limb for gangrene, performed in a few minutes (Fig. 1.1).

Humphry Davy, who is best known for his invention of the safety lamp for coal-miners in the early eighteen hundreds, suggested that nitrous oxide inhalation could be used to deaden surgical pain but the idea was not pursued at the time. Curiously nitrous oxide, and in turn ether, were used for the amusement of the public in America, where parties were held at which the gas or ether vapour was inhaled. In the early part of the nineteenth century it was common for the programme in a British music hall to include an item on the inhalation of nitrous oxide (Fig. 1.2). Both nitrous oxide and ether vapour induced a state similar to alcoholic intoxication which the participants found to be pleasant, and their antics under

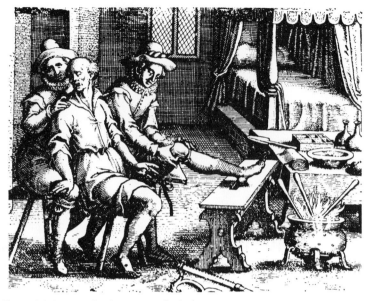

Figure 1.1 An operation in pre-anaesthetic days.

the influence of the drugs were a source of amusement to onlookers. At one party—an 'ether frolic' as it was called—it was noticed
that while under the influence of ether quite severe bruises could be
sustained without the subject being aware of the injury. Similar
observations were made at a session where a young man injured his
leg after breathing nitrous oxide and was again unaware of the
injury. These observations of the protective effects of the agents
against pain led eventually to their being introduced into dental and
surgical practice.

Early demonstrations in America met with varying success but
over the years 1842–1846 further attempts were made and in 1846
ether was successfully used as an anaesthetic for a surgical procedure and the foundations of modern practice were established.

The introduction of new drugs, the development of equipment
with which to administer the drugs and the evolution of safer
methods of administration followed over the next century and,
during the last few decades particularly, the administration of
anaesthetics has passed largely into the hands of doctors specially
trained for this work.

☞ *POSITIVELY THE LAST NIGHT.*

ADELPHI THEATRE

BY AUTHORITY OF THE]   **STRAND.**   [*LORD CHAMBERLAIN*

Notwithstanding the very great Success of M. HENRY's ENTERTAINMENT, it must positively be withdrawn, owing to previous Engagements, after

SATURDAY, JUNE 5, 1824.

THE NITROUS OXIDE, OR

LAUGHING GAS

Will continue to be administered to any of the Audience who may chuse to inhale it; the WONDERS of which were first experienced by

SIR HUMPHREY DAVY,

And the exhilarating Effects it produced, as described by that Gentleman, have been fully evinced during the Period of its Exhibition by M. H. Theatric BURSTS and STARTS à la

KEAN,

By some, **PAS SEULS** or **PIROUETTES** à la

VESTRIS OR *ALBERT*,

Have been commonly performed by others, with **BRAVURAS** to rival

BRAHAM,

And **SCREAMS** of Regret, superior to any ever uttered by

Mrs. HATTON or Mrs. GIBBS,

At the Loss of the Delight, this Gas alone can give, have been of such frequent Occurrence, that many have supposed those highly gifted

PERFORMERS were PRESENT in Disguise.

M. HENRY's ASTONISHING AND MAGNIFICENT DISPLAY OF

Uncommon Illusions, Wonderful Metamorphoses, &c.

Interesting Illustrations in

Experimental Chemistry, Animated Paintings, &c.

IN PARTS I & II of the Entertainment, M. HENRY will exhibit his New and

ASTONISHING ILLUSIONS!

Amazing Combinations, Transformations, &c. &c.

Amongst which will be found

| The THREE WISHES, | The COIN of DIVINATION, | The WONDERFUL FLIGHT, |
| The ENCHANTED FRUIT, | Which answers any Question, | The SAGACIOUS LIVE BIRD, &c. |

PART III:–NOVEL AND INTERESTING

EXPERIMENTS on GAS!!

Amongst which, will be introduced the Inflation and *ASCENT OF A BALLOON* in the Theatre, and

THE LAUGHING GAS.

In the Course of the Evening, M. HENRY will attempt several Melodies, Popular Airs, &c. On that unrivalled Instrument for Sweetness of Tone,

THE MUSICAL GLASSES.

The Evening's Entertainments will conclude with M. HENRY's celebrated

OPTICAL ILLUSIONS

In the Course of which in addition to the STRIKING LIKENESSES of

| Miss STEPHENS, | Miss PATON, | Mr. MACREADY, |
| Miss M. TREE, | Mr. YOUNG, | Mr. KEAN, |

Mr. GRIMALDI, Will be introduced beautiful finished *Portraits* of

King Henry VIII, Anna Boleyn, and Queen Elizabeth.

And likewise

A beautiful Portrait of the immortal SHAKSPEARE,

During the exhibition of which, FAME will be seen to descend and crown him with a Wreath of Laurel, being one of the finest Optic Illusions ever produced...Previous to which,

THE DANCE OF DEATH!! with a Variety of Laughable Figures, &c. &c.

The Programme, &c. and other Instruments of which M. H's Spectacle is composed, together with the Decorations, &c. are of the most splendid Description.

BOXES, 4s. PIT, 2s. GAL. 1s.   Doors open at Half-past 6, and commence at 7.   HALF PRICE, at Half-past 8.

☞ Box Office open from 10, till 4, where Places may be taken, and a Private Box had Nightly of Mr. CALLAN

Children in Arms cannot be admitted.   No Money returned.   Printed by W. GLINDON Rupert Street Haymarket

Figure 1.2 Handbill advertising the inhalation of nitrous oxide as a music hall entertainment (reproduced by kind permission of the Victoria and Albert Museum).

The impact which the introduction of anaesthesia had on surgery can be judged from the fact that in the years before 1842 about 120 operations were performed each year in the whole of the city of Glasgow. In addition, as previously mentioned, many of these operations lasted only a few minutes so that the operating time represented by the 120 operations was not great. Nevertheless, in those days, Glasgow was regarded by young surgeons as a most desirable centre to attend because of the wide experience which could be obtained by seeing so many operations! One has only to think of the countless thousands of operations carried out safely, painlessly and without haste today to realise what a blessing these chance discoveries have been to mankind.

We have now reached the stage where anaesthetic care is considered to include the preoperative preparation and postoperative supervision of the patient. The actual administration of the anaesthetic in theatre is only one part of the sequence. While the nurse plays an important part at all stages, the anaesthetist has come to rely on her to an ever increasing degree in the preparation of the patient and especially in the supervision of the potentially hazardous postoperative period.

2

Basic concepts

Analgesia means absence of pain and is a term used to describe the state in which pain has been abolished but other sensations remain, and the patient is conscious.

Anaesthesia means absence of all sensation. The term implies that the patient is unconscious and all sensation is lost.

Pathways of pain

When a painful stimulus, such as the cut of a surgeon's knife, is applied to an area of the body impulses are transmitted from the endings of the small nerves present in the area. Thence the impulses pass along to larger nerves formed by the union of groups of these small nerves. In this way the impulses reach the spinal cord and travel along tracts in it until they reach the sensory cortex of the brain where they are appreciated as pain. The pathway is called the sensory pathway and the nerves are called sensory nerves, as they carry sensation to the brain (Fig. 2.1).

The conduction of the painful impulses to the brain from the site of injury may be interrupted at any point between their origin and the cerebral cortex where they are appreciated as pain. They may also be interrupted in a variety of ways. We are concerned here with the use of drugs which do this. Surgeons may also interrupt these impulses by cutting the nerve supply to an area invaded by

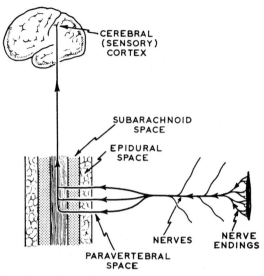

Figure 2.1 The pathway of pain: the course of painful impulses from a wound to the brain is illustrated. The passage of the impulse can be interrupted at any of the sites indicated by the arrows.

an incurable painful tumour or, by dividing a tract in the spinal cord, they may alleviate the pain caused by such a tumour. Tumours themselves may interrupt the passage of impulses along nerves and, of course, injury to the nerve, such as follows some types of fracture for example, has a similar effect. Extreme cold also has an analgesic effect.

EFFECTS OF DRUGS

Drugs may be used to dull pain in two ways.

Local action

Local anaesthetic drugs may be deposited close to the nerves carrying the impulses to the brain. Thus injections may be made at the site of injury, producing the effect by blocking conduction in the nerve endings. Alternatively the drug may be injected around a nerve or group of nerves supplying a region of the body. The drug permeates the nerve and stops conduction of the impulses at that point. This is therefore a local action. It is not known exactly how such a drug produces its effects but certain characteristics of these drugs are known:

Larger (thicker) nerves require stronger solutions to block them compared with fine nerves which may be blocked by relatively dilute solutions.

When a nerve is composed of sensory fibres, motor fibres and branches from the autonomic nervous system, weaker solutions will affect the autonomic branches (affecting arterial pressure, gut motility, etc.), moderate concentrations will block sensory branches, and stronger solutions will be needed to interrupt motor conduction.

Consider a patient who has received extradural (epidural) nerve block for the relief of pain during and after cholecystectomy (see p. 11). A solution of bupivacaine 0.25% will be likely to abolish pain but not the motor nerves to the abdominal and intercostal muscles. A 0.5% solution will cause a motor block; this might be of value in aiding the surgeon's access to the abdomen during the operation but could be an embarrassment to breathing in the postoperative period. Both concentrations can be expected to cause a decrease in arterial pressure.

Centrally acting drugs: general anaesthesia

Instead of attempting to block the passage of the painful impulse to the brain, it is possible to depress the cerebral cortex which receives the impulse so that the pain is either felt with diminished intensity or not felt at all. The drugs which act in this way are of course not brought directly into contact with the cortex by injection in that area, but are carried to the brain in the blood stream. Usually they are administered by way of injection to the blood stream, or by inhalation to the lungs (Fig. 2.2). Again the way in which they produce their effects is not known exactly, but reversible depression of the brain cells occurs. As a rule the more drug that is given the greater the degree of depression produced and the longer will the effects last. During many types of general anaesthesia it is possible to assess the 'depth' of anaesthesia by the presence or absence of certain signs. At a light level of anaesthesia the patient is unconscious but moves, often in an exaggerated fashion, in response to a

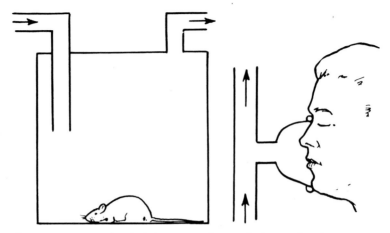

Figure 2.2 Two examples of inhalation anaesthesia. In both cases the subject breathes in a gaseous environment containing anaesthetics. Clearly the box method would be unsuitable for the patient undergoing surgery! The anaesthetic circuit is, nevertheless, only a sophisticated means of isolating the environment from which the patient breathes.

stimulus such as an incision of skin. The cough and, sometimes, the swallowing reflex are present. At a deeper level suitable for surgery there is no movement in response to stimulation and the cough and swallowing reflexes are abolished (obtunded). At excessively deep levels of anaesthesia the function of respiratory muscles is impaired and there is a risk of death from respiratory failure. It is of interest to note that a similar assessment of unconsciousness is used in the management of patients in coma from whatever cause.

General anaesthesia for many types of major surgery involves the use of muscle relaxant drugs (p. 18) and a consequent need to ventilate the lungs artificially. In these circumstances the signs of anaesthesia described above do not apply and great skill is required to be sure that the patient is, in fact, anaesthetised adequately even although the operation may appear to be proceeding uneventfully. Failure to recognise an insufficient depth of anaesthesia in these circumstances results in the notorious problem of 'awareness during surgery'.

3

Methods of analgesia and anaesthesia

REGIONAL OR LOCAL ANALGESIA

Topical application (Fig. 3.1)

Local analgesic solutions may be painted or sprayed on to mucous membranes or open wounds to lessen or abolish sensation. This method is commonly used in the nose, throat and bronchial tree as a preparation for endoscopy. The dose of drug must be measured carefully as absorption through a mucous membrane can be very rapid and toxic reactions may occur. The method is ineffective where the solution is applied to unbroken skin as the drug is not absorbed and does not reach nerve endings.

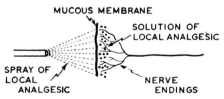

Figure 3.1 Topical application.

Local infiltration (Fig. 3.2)

Injection of a dilute analgesic solution in the area of operation will block the perception of pain at the level of the nerve endings. This is

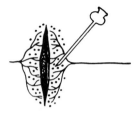

Figure 3.2 Local infiltration.

perhaps the simplest method of analgesia and is widely used for minor surgical operations, including the suture of skin lacerations. If it is restricted to this type of work it is a safe procedure and has little in the way of after-effects so that the patient is able to eat, drink and return home shortly after operation. The method can be used for more extensive operations but in such cases larger doses of the drugs are used; and thus side-effects are more likely and the safety margin is reduced. Extensive infiltration of a local anaesthetic solution is unpleasant for the patient.

Intravenous injection

A dilute solution of a local analgesic drug may be injected intravenously distal to a tourniquet in a limb previously rendered bloodless. This method, which can be used for operations or manipulations on the limbs, is simple to use and normally has few side-effects (see p. 38).

Nerve blocks (Fig. 3.3)

If we know the route taken by the main nerves which supply the area of an operation we can inject local analgesic solution close to the nerves. In this way it is possible with a small number of injections

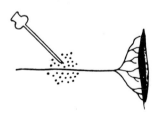

Figure 3.3 Regional nerve block.

to produce analgesia over a wide area. This is achieved by using quite small doses of the drugs and is less painful than widespread infiltration. Sometimes when it is intended to operate within the abdomen under local anaesthesia the autonomic fibres must be blocked. Some pain fibres find their way to the spinal cord using the pathways of the autonomic nerve supply. In addition blockade of fibres controlling blood vessel size may be beneficial by reducing arterial pressure in, and improving venous drainage from, the site of operation; this *deliberate hypotension* may greatly reduce blood loss at operation and avoid or minimise the need for blood transfusion with its attendant hazards. Paravertebral extradural and spinal nerve block can all produce a degree of autonomic block.

Paravertebral block (Fig. 3.4)

In this method of analgesia the nerves are blocked close to the vertebrae (para = beside) before the sympathetic branch has left the main nerve. This technique can be used for surgical procedures inside the abdomen but as it involves multiple injections it is not popular for this type of case. Its use nowadays is usually restricted to the blocking of a few nerves such as the supply to a leg, to produce a vasodilation in vascular disease (lumbar sympathetic nerve block).

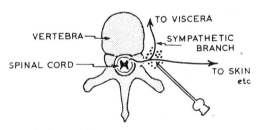

Figure 3.4 Paravertebral nerve block.

Epidural (extradural) nerve block or analgesia (Fig. 3.5)

This consists of the injection of a local analgesic solution into the space between the outer and inner layers of the dura mater. The outer dura acts as a lining for the bony spinal canal. The inner layer is closely adherent to the arachnoid mater to produce the so-called dura-arachnoid membrane. The epidural space contains fat tissue,

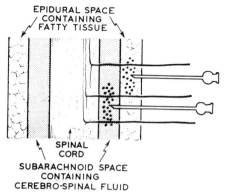

EPIDURAL SPACE
CONTAINING
FATTY TISSUE

SPINAL
CORD

SUBARACHNOID SPACE
CONTAINING
CEREBRO-SPINAL FLUID

Figure 3.5 Epidural and spinal analgesia: the diagram illustrates the two sites at which the analgesic solution is deposited, following introduction of the needle through the intervertebral space.

the epidural veins in a plexus and the segmental nerve routes to and from the spinal cord. In the epidural space the solution can travel up and down the spinal canal depending on the site of injection, the volume injected and the position of the patient; with only one injection many nerve routes can be bathed in the local anaesthetic solution and analgesia of a wide area can be produced. Injections may be made through a suitable needle or a catheter may be introduced and repeated injections can be given through it during a prolonged operation and in the postoperative period (continuous epidural analgesia). This type of analgesia is of use in patients with chronic lung disease where general anaesthesia may be difficult or the use of potent narcotic analgesics such as morphine is undesirable. This type of analgesia is very popular for pain relief in labour and is becoming popular in some centres for Caesarean section.

Spinal (subarachnoid) nerve block or analgesia

This is a method by which widespread analgesia is produced by depositing local anaesthetic solution in the cerebrospinal fluid in the subarachnoid space. It produces good analgesia, excellent muscle relaxation and a contracted bowel making access to the abdomen easy. The decrease in arterial pressure which occurs reduces surgical haemorrhage. In most patients subarachnoid nerve block is easier to perform than epidural nerve block. At present it is gaining popularity in Britain having been out of favour for almost 30 years, but throughout that time the method has been widely used in many countries of the world. Complications of the technique include headache which may be severe and can persist for several days.

Whenever local analgesia is practised, particularly nerve block techniques, it is essential to prepare for the injection with the same care as would be given before laparotomy. For subarachnoid analgesia it is desirable to use a fine gauge needle. This reduces the size of the hole in the dura-arachnoid and is thought to reduce the leakage of cerebral-spinal fluid and thus the incidence of post-spinal headache.

Drugs used for regional analgesia

Many drugs may be used for these techniques, the commonest being lignocaine (Xylocaine) and bupivacaine (Marcain). Others available include prilocaine (Citanest), mepivacaine (Carbocaine) and etidocaine (Duranest). Amethocaine (Decicain) is commonly used as a lozenge to anaesthetise the mouth and pharynx as a prelude to bronchoscopy, oesophagoscopy, etc. Cinchocaine (Nupercaine) is very popular for spinal analgesia. All the drugs interrupt the passage of impulses along the nerve fibres; the stronger the concentration the larger the diameter of nerve fibre which can be blocked.

Under most circumstances part of the local anaesthetic drug injected is absorbed to the blood stream causing a feeling of warmth and dizziness from vasodilation and a decrease in arterial pressure. Toxic effects include circulatory collapse and convulsions. The risk of toxicity increases as the blood concentration increases. This is why it is important to check that a local anaesthetic solution is not being injected directly to a blood vessel by accident.

The nurse handling local anaesthetic drugs must check carefully that she gives the doctor exactly what is asked for and must ensure, for spinal and epidural analgesia particularly, that adequate sterilisation of the drugs or ampoules has been carried out. Further details of the care of local analgesic solutions are given in Chapter 6.

GENERAL ANAESTHESIA

General anaesthesia involving loss of consciousness during surgery is the method used for most operations. We can consider anaesthesia as being composed of three parts: hypnosis or sleep, analgesia or the suppression of reflex responses to painful stimuli, and muscle relaxation.

The concept of 'balanced anaesthesia'

It is possible to achieve all the above effects with one or two inhaled drugs, for example halothane in a mixture of nitrous oxide in oxygen. Frequently however it is desirable, from the point of view of the patient's comfort or the ease of surgery, to use a combination of several drugs (inhalation and intravenous) in doses 'balanced' to give the best combination of effects.

Sleep may be induced by intravenous injection of a suitable drug, commonly thiopentone, but may also be induced by inhalation of gases or vapours. The injection is more pleasant for the patient. Sleep is normally maintained by inhalation of nitrous oxide in oxygen frequently supplemented by one of the volatile anaesthetics. It may also be maintained by intermittent or continuous infusion of an intravenous anaesthetic.

Analgesia is normally obtained by the inhalation of nitrous oxide (with oxygen) supplemented by a volatile anaesthetic when necessary or by intravenous injection of a suitable narcotic.

Muscle relaxation of greater or lesser degree is required for most surgical procedures and is usually obtained by injection of specific muscle relaxants. The potent inhalation anaesthetics such as halothane, enflurane or diethyl-ether cause the muscles to relax but the quality of relaxation is not usually sufficient for operations within the abdominal cavity. Sometimes the regional methods described above can be combined with general anaesthesia; local anaesthetic blockade of the motor nerve supply to muscles produces profound relaxation.

Routes of administration

All general anaesthetic agents exert their effects on the brain, to which they are carried in the blood. They reach the blood in one of three ways:

Intravenous injection is the most direct route and it allows the anaesthetist to deliver quickly and accurately a given dose of a drug to the patient. Its very ease, however, makes it a potentially dangerous method and in unskilled hands deaths have been caused by giving an overdose. It is the normal route of administration of the drugs used to commence (induce) anaesthesia, and it is the route of administration of the muscle relaxants and analgesics, such as pethidine, morphine or fentanyl.

Inhalation of vapours or gases enables them to pass via the alveoli into the pulmonary circulation and thus to the arteries and brain. This method is more time consuming and may be unpleasant for all concerned. Because induction is slower, overdosage is less likely and in unskilled hands it is the safest method of producing anaesthesia. It is almost universally used as part of the technique of maintaining sleep and analgesia, the gases and vapours being given in this way continuously throughout the operation.

Intramuscular injection. This route is uncommon in the provision of anaesthesia, as opposed to analgesia. It is used occasionally in children, notable for the administration of ketamine (see later).

Rectal injection of agents used to be popular. A variety of drugs including thiopentone and diethyl-ether ('ether') have been given in this way. These methods have been almost totally abandoned.

DRUGS USED FOR GENERAL ANAESTHESIA

Intravenous agents

The barbiturates remain the most popular drugs for inducing anaesthesia, principally thiopentone and to a lesser extent metho- hexitone. These drugs are not analgesics and are not used as the sole anaesthetic unless for very short procedures. After adminis- tration they are partly redistributed in the body and slowly excreted so that the patient may still be slightly groggy for some time after regaining consciousness.

Althesin is a mixture of two steroid derivatives (Alphaxolone and Alphadolone), both devoid of hormonal activity. Induction with Althesin is fairly rapid and recovery is said to be more pleasant than after barbiturates. In addition the safety margin is high and the drug is non-irritant. Side-effects are few unless large doses are given. Because the drug is metabolised rapidly supplementary doses can be given without a serious risk of Althesin accumulating within the tissue. Althesin has been used as part of one method of *total intravenous anaesthesia.* Althesin may induce an allergic reaction particularly if it has been given on a recent previous occasion.

Propanidid (Epontol) is a non-barbiturate agent which may be used where rapid recovery is particularly desirable. Its popularity has declined because of anxiety about allergic reactions.

Ketamine (Ketalar). This drug is a powerful analgesic and may be given to induce anaesthesia or to produce a state of dissociation short of unconsciousness, with preservation of protective reflexes (coughing and swallowing). It can cause arterial hypertension which may be an advantage in patients suffering from haemorrhagic shock. Vivid dreams or hallucinations may occur during recovery but these can be virtually abolished by the use of sedative pre-medication. Unexpected movement of the patient during a delicate operation may be troublesome unless the ketamine anaesthesia is supplemented with other anaesthetic drugs.

In patients with bad facial burns or on other occasions where an airway may be difficult to maintain, and in cardiac catheterisation, ketamine has been found useful. Side-effects appear to be less in children in whom the drug finds its main application. It may be given intramuscularly if required, or if venepuncture is undesirable or impractical.

Etomidate (Hypnomidate) has been introduced in a number of European countries as an intravenous anaesthetic. It is very rapidly metabolised in the body so that the effect of one injection is brief and it is possible to give a continuous infusion of the drug without accumulation in the tissues or a prolonged hangover effect. Some patients experience pain on injection of Etomidate and this is an obvious disadvantage.

Benzodiazepines. This group of drugs, used mainly as tranquillisers, includes several compounds which may be given intravenously to induce anaesthesia. Diazepam (Valium) is the best known example. On some occasions, even after large doses, the patients do not appear to lose consciousness but may readily accept an inhalation anaesthetic. Diazepam has muscle relaxant properties which make it valuable in the control of epilepsy or tetanus. Benzodiazepines are commonly given as premedicants for anaesthesia and as part of the preparation of a patient for procedures which are to be performed under regional analgesia.

Neuroleptanalgesia. The combination of a neuroleptic drug, which makes the patient indifferent to his surroundings, and a potent analgesic may be used to induce anaesthesia. This is described more fully in Chapter 6.

GASES AND VOLATILE ANAESTHETICS

Gases

Oxygen is, of course, vital to life and is administered during every anaesthetic, either in the form of air or more frequently in controlled proportions in higher concentrations than the 21% normally found in air.

Nitrous oxide is administered with oxygen during most anaesthetics. It is a weak anaesthetic but recovery from it is very rapid. Nitrous oxide is a powerful analgesic and is given in concentrations of up to 50% with oxygen for this purpose. The only other anaesthetic which exists as a gas, as distinct from a vapour, is *cyclopropane*, a very powerful but expensive and explosive agent. Although there are a few enthusiasts for cyclopropane the drug is not widely used.

Volatile liquid anaesthetics

These form a large group and the selection of any one is often a matter of personal preference.

Halothane (Fluothane) is used most often. It is a potent drug but its availability in the last 25 years has contributed greatly to the safety and versatility of anaesthesia. Recovery from halothane is relatively pleasant and rapid. Rare reports of liver damage, alleged to have been caused by halothane, have caused great controversy but the drug continues to be popular.

Enflurane (Ethrane) has a range of properties not unlike those of halothane but it is several times more expensive at present. It is sometimes preferred to halothane in circumstances in which the risk of halothane-induced liver damage is thought to be increased (obesity, previous recent exposure to halothane).

Trichloroethylene (Trilene) is used occasionally as an anaesthetic. It has profound analgesic properties and is used in subanaesthetic concentrations for pain relief in labour.

Methoxyflurane (Penthrane) is also a potent analgesic and may be used for this purpose. It is not very popular as an anaesthetic on account of its slow excretion and recovery and a risk of kidney damage when large doses of the drug are given.

Diethyl-ether (often called simply 'anaesthetic ether') is inflammable in air and explosive when the oxygen concentration of the gas mixture is greater than that in air. Thus ether cannot be used in the presence of surgical diathermy. The uptake of ether is relatively slow and the recovery from ether anaesthesia may be prolonged. Added to these disadvantages ether anaesthesia is associated with a high frequency of vomiting in the postoperative period. In spite of these unwanted effects ether has an established reputation as a relatively safe anaesthetic particularly where the administrator is relatively inexperienced. It is for this reason, plus the fact that ether is relatively inexpensive, that the drug is still widely used in many countries of the world although the specialist anaesthetist would be more likely to select one of the volatile anaesthetics listed above.

Chloroform although one of the traditional anaesthetics is rarely used nowadays. It has a reputation—which some authorities think is undeserved—for causing liver damage and sudden circulatory arrest. Apart from these disadvantages chloroform is in many respects similar in its effects to halothane which has largely superceded it.

NON-VOLATILE ANALGESICS

These may be administered during the course of an anaesthetic as an alternative to the use of the volatile agents. Many drugs have been used for this purpose: morphine, pethidine, phenoperidine, fentanyl, pentazocine, buprenorphine, and many other less well known drugs. The use of analgesics, given in this way, has the advantage that the patient awakens free from pain but may be more drowsy for some time after operation than would be the case where a volatile anaesthetic had been given. These drugs are also more likely to cause inadvertent respiratory depression.

NEUROMUSCULAR BLOCKERS

These drugs act at the junction between the nerve and muscle and prevent transmission of the impulse which would cause the muscle to contract. In this way temporary muscle paralysis is produced. The drugs used are divided into two groups: the 'competitive' agents, tubocurarine (Curare, Tubarine), alcuronium (Alloferin), pancuronium (Pavulon), gallamine (Flaxedil) and fazqdinium (Fazqdon) compete with acetylcholine, the chemical transmitter released at nerve endings, for the receptors on the muscle (Fig. 3.6). The 'depolarising' drugs, suxamethonium (Scoline) and

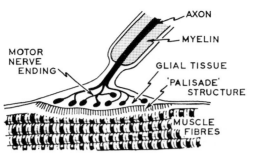

Figure 3.6 The myoneural junction. The 'palisade' structure is the site at which acetylcholine, released from the motor nerve endings, acts upon the muscle fibres to cause contraction.

suxethonium (Brevidil E) mimic acetylcholine's action to the extent that they cause depolarisation of the muscle which appears as contraction or fine muscle twitching fasciculation before paralysis ensues.

The choice of neuromuscular blocking drug is influenced by several factors, the important ones being the duration of action and the likelihood of unwanted side-effects. Pancuronium and tubocurarine, for example, have a longer duration of action than gallamine. Pancuronium is likely to cause a small increase in heart rate and arterial pressure whereas tubocurarine is likely to cause a reduction in arterial pressure. Gallamine causes marked increases in heart rate and is excreted exclusively by the kidney so that it would be unsuitable for patients with renal failure. Suxamethonium has a very short duration of action but can cause marked slowing of the heart in patients with extensive tissue damage such as might occur after severe burns.

The action of the depolarising neuromuscular blocking drugs is antagonised by neostigmine (Prostigmin) and is routinely given at the end of an operation in which these drugs have been used. Neostigmine may have undesired effects of its own including excessive salivation. These unwanted effects are minimised by the injection of atropine which is usually given in combination with neostigmine. There is no available antidote to suxamethonium and suxethonium.

Toxicity of anaesthetic gases and vapours

There has been a great deal of research into the potential of the volatile agents to cause damage to organs. The possibility of liver damage from halothane and chloroform has been mentioned already as has the risk of kidney damage from methoxyflurane. In the last 10 years there has been much concern that trace concentrations of volatile and gaseous anaesthetics in the environment of the operating theatre might be associated with a risk to operating theatre personnel. Particular interest has focused on the possibility that a pregnant woman exposed to such an environment in the early months of pregnancy might have an increased risk of spontaneous abortion and of congenital abnormality in a live-born child. These problems continue to attract the interest of reseachers but the present best opinions suggest (and the matter has not been proved definitely) that the risk can be minimised by the use of appropriate scavenging apparatus which ducts the patient's exhaled gas to the outside of the hospital building. Irrespective of these specific fears about health it is probably good hygiene to duct away the anaesthetic gases and to avoid breathing in the direct line of a patient's exhaled gas during the early period of recovery from anaesthesia. It follows, of course, that there should be a careful code of discipline in the operating theatre to avoid accidental spillage of volatile anaesthestics.

4

Preparation of the patient for anaesthesia

Written permission for operation and anaesthesia

Written permission for anaesthesia must always be obtained. In Britain an individual of 16 years of age or over may give consent for treatment without the authority of a parent or guardian, provided he is capable of understanding what this treatment involves. The consent of a parent or guardian should, however, be obtained where the patient is under the age of 16. In an emergency every reasonable effort should be made to obtain written consent but where the patient is, for example, unconscious or relatives are not readily available, essential treatment should not be withheld.

The purpose of the operation should be explained to the patient or parent. Whenever possible the consent form should be kept in the patient's record folder and be checked by the anaesthetist.

Identification of patients

It is vitally important that all patients going to theatre should bear adequate means of identification. The possibility of operating on the wrong patient, or of carrying out the wrong operation, is increased when the staff involved in the preparations for the operation, in the ward or theatre, are unfamiliar with the patient. Identification is usually accomplished by attaching to the patient's wrist a label which bears his or her name, age and address. This

21

label should be attached to the patient soon after admission to hospital; patients may visit other parts of the hospital for investigations, sometimes under anaesthesia, before undergoing the operation for which they were admitted. Care must also be taken to ensure that all concerned know what operation is proposed and, where an operation may be performed on either side, for example ligation of varicose veins or herniorrhaphy, it is clearly understood which side is to be operated on. It is therefore wise to mark the site and side of operation and to check that the side is correct with each patient immediately before the induction of anaesthesia.

Psychological preparation

Psychological preparation for what is, in most cases, an ordeal is of great importance. Here a thoughtful nurse can be invaluable. For most patients an operation is a major ordeal—and for many it is an unfamiliar experience. The nurse has an important role in the psychological preparation which can contribute greatly to the patient's mental and physical wellbeing. The patient should be protected from the Job's comforters who are to be found in most wards; contact with sensible patients who are recovering from surgery can be particularly reassuring. In addition to these measures, the nurse on her rounds should find time to explain something of the hospital routine to those in her charge and indicate briefly what lies ahead. Patients can be spared unnecessary worry if they are told about the events leading to their transfer to the operating theatre and reassured that they will not be taken into theatre awake. Many patients still fear that the induction of anaesthesia is associated with an evil smelling mask and are relieved to hear that in modern practice this is replaced by an almost painless injection. One of the greatest fears is the fear of the unknown and a few words of explanation and advice from a thoughtful nurse are worth much sedation from a doctor. Many patients justifiably complain that they are treated as children, being told little of what is going to happen to them.

Smoking

Smoking is a contributory factor in postoperative pulmonary complications. Stopping smoking for a week or more before surgery is likely to lessen the risk of complications. For those who have been unable to do that, however, it is arguable if prevention of smoking on the night before operation (as is sometimes expected by nurses and anaesthetists) confers any nett benefit. It is unlikely that the bronchial tree would improve much from the chronic effects of smoking and the patient may be denied a means of solace at a time of stress.

Emptying the stomach

Perhaps the most important single precaution which can be taken in preparing a patient for anaesthesia is to ensure that the stomach is empty. Of the small number of deaths which can be attributed to anaesthesia a significance proportion are caused by vomiting or regurgitation of stomach contents with inhalation of vomitus to the lungs. Vomiting is an active process which is obvious to the onlooker but regurgitation is a silent emptying of the stomach into the pharynx which may take place at any time during anaesthesia and may pass unnoticed. For this reason, among others, prevention is of the utmost importance.

Elective operation. Food, fluids and sweets should be withheld for at least 4 hours before the time of the operation. In addition, it is important to explain to the patient why this is being done and to point out to him that he must not eat or drink from his own supplies. If in doubt, these supplies should be removed from the bedside locker.

Emergency operations. Sometimes it may be possible to delay the operation until the required 4 hours from the time the meal was consumed have passed. This is not always feasible and, in some cases (see below), is not a sufficient guarantee that the stomach will be empty. Active steps can be taken to empty the stomach, either by the use of a large-bore stomach tube or by the administration of an emetic such as apomorphine. Normally, a large-bore stomach tube is used when food has been consumed and lavage may further help to remove it. A Ryle's tube has a too narrow bore to be of any value for gastric emptying.

Apomorphine is only occasionally used although it is a very effective emetic. The profuse salivation and severe bradycardia which accompany its use are very unpleasant for the patient.

The stomach should be emptied when:

A meal has been consumed less than 4 hours before operation.

There is reason to believe that the normal emptying time of the stomach may be prolonged, for example, in pregnancy, or if an injury has been sustained shortly after a meal. It is common for a patient who has suffered an injury to a limb, within an hour or so of a meal, to have a full stomach 10 or more hours later.

Patients with intestinal obstruction or peritonitis may have excessive gastric secretion or retrograde filling of the stomach from the bowel and should always be considered at risk from vomiting or regurgitation.

Once a stomach tube has been passed, the stomach content should be aspirated and this aspiration should be repeated before the patient is taken to the anaesthetic room. The precaution of ensuring that the stomach is empty must be taken before any but the most trivial local analgesics. After spinal and epidural analgesia a patient may vomit and be unable to clear his pharynx. Although the patients are usually conscious after these procedures they may fall asleep from time to time during the operation. If this happens and the stomach is manipulated by the surgeon causing regurgitation, inhalation of gastric contents may take place. In addition, when the abdomen is opened and retractors are in place, the normal cough mechanism is impaired. After other forms of local analgesia, there is always a risk of a toxic reaction, for example a convulsion which would require thiopentone or a relaxant to control it. Here the risk of regurgitation is obvious. A stomach tube inserted to prevent regurgitation should be left in position without a spiggot as a further aid to gastric drainage and decompression. The end of the tube may be connected to an appropriate suction apparatus or be allowed to drain to a polythene bag.

Antacid therapy

One of the complications associated with vomiting or regurgitation of stomach contents during anaesthesia is the acid aspiration syndrome or Mendelson's syndrome. The patient develops severe bronchospasm and circulatory collapse and the condition may be rapidly fatal. These changes are a result of the acidity of the inhaled stomach content and may be minimised by giving an antacid solution, such as 15 ml magnesium trisilicate, by mouth half an hour preoperatively. Such a regimen is of particular value in obstetric patients (see Ch. 7). Metoclopramide (Maxolon) promotes gastric emptying to the duodenum while cimetidine (Tagomet) reduces acid production by the stomach. Both drugs have their advocates for reducing the risk of regurgitation and pulmonary aspiration respectively.

Emptying the bladder and bowel

The bladder and bowel should be emptied. This precaution should be observed before every anaesthetic, although the method used will vary. Thus, before a major gynaecological operation, it is usual to empty the bladder by catheter and before a major bowel operation an enema is often given. It is also important that the out-patient should be directed to a toilet before even the most trivial procedure, lest he soil his clothes after induction of anaesthesia adding unnecessary discomfort to his journey home. The urine should always be tested for common abnormal constituents (sugar, ketone bodies, albumen) and the result reported.

SPECIAL CASES

It is not possible to consider all the special preoperative preparations for the different types of patient or operation and in any case these will vary from one hospital to another. Some of the more common are given below.

Where the patient has an acute respiratory infection, the operation should be postponed if possible. The likelihood of postoperative chest complications is increased when an anaesthetic is given during the first 3 to 4 days of a common cold—the so-called invasive period. If the operation cannot be delayed an antibiotic may be given to reduce the danger of secondary bacterial invasion.

Patients with a chronic respiratory condition should, if possible, be operated on during a period of remission, usually in the spring and summer. Physiotherapy, in the form of breathing exercises, should be given preoperatively and may usefully be combined with administrations of bronchodilator drugs. If the sputum is infected, appropriate chemotherapy should be given.

Where the patient is found to be anaemic it may be appropriate to institute iron therapy with a view to undertaking the operation when the haemoglobin concentration has reached acceptable levels. If this is not possible then the patient may be given blood or preferably concentrated red cells. The precise course of management, however, will be the result of weighing a number of factors.

The benefits of blood transfusion have to be set against the risks of overloading the circulation in a patient with heart disease. Some patients with chronic anaemia, notably those with chronic renal failure, are able to alter the manner in which oxygen is transported by the blood so as to compensate for marked reductions in haemoglobin concentration.

The presence of mild uncomplicated hypertension is not regarded as a contraindication to a carefully given anaesthetic. In many patients it may be a sign of preoperative anxiety and the blood pressure returns to normal postoperatively. If in doubt selected cases may be treated by rest in bed and mild sedation for a few days.

More severe hypertension presents a difficult problem. Some patients will benefit from antihypertensive therapy, adjusted as necessary for the period of operation. An elective operation may be postponed until the patient is on a stable regimen.

Cardiac decompensation will necessitate active treatment with diuretics, digitalis, or other appropriate measures.

Diabetes. Patients who are under treatment with long acting insulins or with oral hypoglycaemic drugs, especially chlorpropamide (Diabinese), should be brought under control with soluble insulin on the day before operation. On the day of operation itself a glucose infusion is set up. *Never give glucose orally before operation*. The urine is tested with one of the commercial colour indicator papers and soluble insulin is given subcutaneously on the following scale:

Colour	Treatment
Green	10 units of soluble insulin
Yellow	20 units of soluble insulin
Orange	30 units of soluble insulin

After operation, the regimen is continued, the urine being tested 3-hourly, and only when the patient is stabilised on diet are long-acting agents restarted.

Patients who have received prolonged steroid therapy should be considered as special anaesthetic risks. These drugs can suppress the function of the adrenal gland which plays a part in the patient's response to stress. Anaesthesia, surgery and postoperative complications are considerable stresses for which the patient may be unable to compensate and this must be allowed for when prescribing supplementary steroid therapy. Even if steroid therapy has been discontinued for some time before surgery the patient may still be at risk. The extent to which a patient is able to respond to stress may be determined in the laboratory; in routine practice, however, it is more convenient simply to assume a risk and to give hydrocortisone.

Many patients may be receiving sedative therapy. These drugs may affect the course of anaesthesia in one of two ways. Patients who are receiving phenothiazine derivatives such as chlorpromazine may require very little thiopentone and, indeed, if more than minimal doses of this drug are given, marked arterial hypotension and prolonged recovery may follow. On the other hand, patients who are habituated to alcohol may be very resistant to normal doses of anaesthetic agents and induction may prove difficult in such cases. This is the result of enzyme induction in the liver which results in excessively rapid breakdown of the anaesthetic agents.

The monoamine oxidase inhibitor group of drugs, used in the treatment of depression, may cause severe hypertension, particularly after amphetamine-like drugs. Abnormal reactions to narcotics, such as hypotension, hypertension and hyperpyrexia, may occur also. Such drugs may be associated with delayed recovery of consciousness after general anaesthesia, and with liver damage.

Antihypertensive agents. Patients receiving such therapy present a problem to the anaesthetist. If such a patient is anaesthetised, a profound reduction in arterial pressure, which may not respond to vasopressor therapy, may be encountered. If, on the other hand, antihypertensive therapy is discontinued, the patient is submitted to surgery with an increased strain on his heart. Special mention should be made of methyldopa, a commonly used antihypertensive agent. As this drug is unlikely to interfere with the drugs which will be used during anaesthesia and with the resuscitative measures likely to be employed, the present recommendation is that it should not be discontinued in anticipation of anaesthesia and surgery.

Many patients who are being treated for hypertension may be receiving diuretics and this may result in potassium depletion with alteration in the response to muscle relaxant drugs. It is important to measure the serum potassium concentration before operation.

Beta adrenergic blocking drugs (propranolol, practolol). These drugs are employed in the treatment of a variety of conditions, notably angina. There has been considerable controversy about the advisability of continuing this therapy in patients undergoing anaesthesia and surgery. The current view is that therapy should be maintained.

Antibiotics in large doses may potentiate the drugs such as curare and pancuronium. All 'mycin' drugs such as neomycin and streptomycin produce this effect.

Oral contraceptives may inhibit the breakdown of pethidine in the body. Although they may increase the incidence of venous thrombosis during and after operation, current opinion is opposed to stopping therapy on the grounds that the adverse effects may take many weeks to disappear. Subcutaneous heparin therapy (5000 units) should be given to reduce the risk of thrombosis.

Where examination reveals alteration in the plasma proteins or unsatisfactory electrolyte concentrations, intravenous therapy should be commenced to ensure that these deficiencies are remedied before anaesthesia and operation.

Final checking

When sedative premedication has been given the patient should not sit up unless there is an obvious need to do so, because there is an increased risk of fainting. The patient should put on the theatre gown before premedication. Premedicated patients should be allowed to lie quietly in an area where they may be supervised in case there is an unexpected drug reaction such as confusion, respiratory depression or circulatory collapse.

Before leaving the ward, the nurse should give the patient a final check and remove:

False teeth, a watch, wig or glass eye or contact lenses lest these are damaged in theatre.

An engagement ring and, in some cases, a wedding ring where the fingers may swell (as in wrist fractures).

Hairpins, lest they injure the head (or the anaesthetist's hand!).

Make-up and lipstick. The latter precaution allows the anaesthetist to look for cyanosis in the lips, cheeks and nail beds, the sites at which it is most easily recognised.

Theatre gowns should allow easy access to all parts of the patient's body and should be easily removable after anaesthesia has commenced.

The nurse should ensure:

That the patient has adequate pillows and blankets to keep him comfortable and warm on his journey to the anaesthetic room. Many patients are uncomfortable lying flat with only one pillow and some are cold when transferred from bed. Pillows should be firm but malleable; this is important in positioning the head for laryngoscopy and tracheal intubation. Most anaesthetists regard foam rubber pillows as quite unsuitable (and they are not particularly comfortable for the patient in any case).

That the pillow and the patient's head rest *on* the stretcher (Fig. 4.1). If the pillow is placed beyond the end of the stretcher, when the unconscious patient is lifted, the head falls and serious injury may result (Fig. 4.2). Patients have died from broken necks in this way.

The patient's name, age, disease, and on what side the operation is to be carried out.

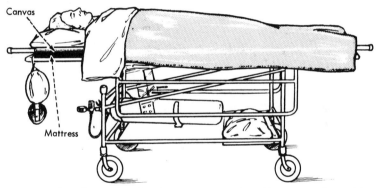

Figure 4.1 The pillow is placed *on* the canvas, *not* on the rubber mattress beyond the end of the canvas.

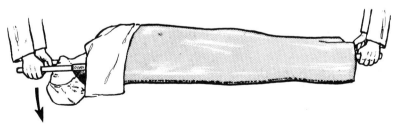

Figure 4.2 Here a patient, placed on an incorrectly set trolley, has been lifted. The pillow has fallen and the unsupported head is dangerously hyperextended.

That the identity label with this information is in place.
That the patient's X-rays and case sheet accompany him.

The nurse should know:
What treatment has been ordered and carried out, what drugs have been given, and the time and route of their administration. It is equally important that, if any drug or treatment has been ordered and not given or carried out, for whatever reason, this should be reported to the anaesthetist. It is almost always possible to remedy an omission before anaesthesia is induced but an unrecognised or undisclosed omission may cost the patient his life!

The use of special checklists to be completed at various stages of preparation by the appropriate persons helps to ensure that nothing has been overlooked. Note should also be made of any infirmity, distress or limitation of limb movement which may not be immediately obvious to the theatre staff.

5

Premedication

Premedication may be given for three reasons:
1. To relieve anxiety. This may include pain relief.
2. To abolish or reduce undesirable parasympathetic activity.
3. To reduce postoperative vomiting.

The relief of anxiety (sedation) is the most important function of premedication. When pain is present before operation, anxiety may be relieved by alleviating the pain. In other cases, psychic sedation is required.

Reassurance and simple explanations to the patient can save much in the way of drugs. Many patients will benefit from a simple explanation of hospital routine. They will appreciate being told that on the night before operation they will receive a hypnotic. They will also appreciate being told that, before going to theatre, pre-anaesthetic sedatives will be given so that they will approach the anaesthetic room with minimal anxiety. Many who have had previous surgery and have unpleasant memories of an inhalation induction will appreciate the promise of an intravenous induction. Despite the advent of medical television programmes, many patients know little of the routine of a surgical ward or theatre and their greatest fear is of the unknown.

While this psychological preparation is helpful, it is seldom in itself adequate to relieve anxiety and some form of sedative drug is normally given.

In very nervous patients, a mild sedative may be given for a few days before admission or soon after admission.

Parasympathetic overactivity during anaesthesia may be manifest as bradycardia, excessive secretion of saliva and bronchial mucus, or as broncho-constriction. Although, with the use of modern agents, irritation of the bronchi with excessive secretion is less common, and the routine use of a belladonna derivative is now being questioned, many anaesthetists still include such a drug in a premedicant mixture. The drugs used commonly are atropine sulphate or hyoscine hydrobromide (Scopolamine).

Atropine in appropriate dosage may be given to patients of all ages but has no sedative properties. *Hyoscine* provides welcome amnesia, the patient remembering little of what has happened. Its disadvantages are that it has no vagolytic action and, indeed, may cause slight slowing of the heart. In older patients, hyoscine may cause restlessness and confusion and its use is usually restricted to patients under the age of 60.

Often, atropine or hyoscine is incorporated in the premedication given about 1 hour before surgery. However, some anaesthestists, to avoid causing the patient to have a dry mouth during this period, omit the belladonna derivative from the original injection and inject it intravenously at the time of induction.

The choice of sedation used in the immediate preoperative period is determined by the general health of the patient, the nature of the operation and anaesthetic, and the preferences of the anaesthetist. For example, although the opiates are probably the most widely used premedicants in most hospitals their ability to cause respiratory depression might render them inappropriate for a patient with advanced chronic lung disease who was about to undergo an endoscopic procedure, the anticipation of which did not appear to be causing him undue distress. The patient undergoing inguinal herniorrhaphy with spinal anaesthesia might be better served by a benzodiazepine premedicant as opposed to morphine which might make him sick; on the other hand the opiates and other narcotic drugs can have an important effect in lessening the requirements for the drugs used during the anaesthetic itself. There is a wide range of drugs from which the choice of a preoperative sedative can be made. The nurse who is in contact with several anaesthetists might be excused for believing that the choice of compound was apparently random. Although there are differing practices, and strongly held views as to what constitutes the correct approach most anaesthetists select premedicant drugs with great care since they will compliment their particular method of anaesthesia in a given patient.

The opiates. Morphine and allied drugs are still widely used in premedication despite the many other drugs which are available. They produce analgesia, psychic sedation and a state of euphoria which is very welcome before an operation. The opiates are non-irritant solutions and may be injected subcutaneously or intramuscularly. The main disadvantages are that they produce a high incidence of postoperative vomiting, 30–40%, and are respiratory depressants.

Morphine sulphate is normally given in a dose of 0.2 mg kg^{-1} to a maximum of 15 mg; morphine is derived from opium. Papaveretum (Omnopon) is a mixture of opium derivatives 60% being morphine. Papaveretum is administered in a dose of 0.3 mg kg^{-1} to a maximum of 20 mg. It is considered less liable to produce nausea and vomiting, because of the presence of some of the other opium derivatives, but this is doubtful. Many of the disadvantages of the opiates such as respiratory depression and vomiting occur only when the dose given is too large for a particular patient.

Pethidine hydrochloride was introduced as a substitute for morphine. It was claimed originally that it produced less respiratory depression and less nausea and vomiting than did the opiates. There is now reason to doubt these claims. Pethidine is a poorer sedative and produces less euphoria than the opiates. Given in equi-analgesic dosage the side-effects are probably similar to those found after the use of morphine and the sedative properties are much less. The dose for premedication in an adult is usually in the range of 50–100 mg i.m.

Pethidine is claimed to have a relaxing effect on the muscles of the bronchial tree and may be useful in patients in whom bronchospasm is present or suspected. It is also widely used in obstetric practice because it has a dilating effect on the cervix during labour.

The use of analgesic agents in premedication has been questioned because, it is claimed, when they are administered to pain-free anxious patients they may fail to relieve anxiety and produce a state of confusion or dysphoria instead. It is also claimed that if narcotics are omitted from premedication, but given during or after anaesthesia when the patient is in pain, the incidence of emetic sequelae is reduced. Thus attention has been directed towards other groups of drugs.

The benzodiazepines. This group of drugs is an important class of compound used as hypnotic sedatives and anxiolytics. Although some are marketed specifically for their hypnotic effect as a general rule it can be said that these compounds have a sedative or anxiolytic effect in low dosage and a hypnotic effect in high dosage. Chlordiazepoxide (Librium) is a well-known anxiolytic but is little used in anaesthetic practice. Diazepam (Valium) has been widely used in premedication given either orally or by intravenous injection; injection into the muscle is painful and is best avoided. Temazepam (Normison) and flurazepam (Dalmane) both enjoy popularity as hypnotics and have been used as premedicants also. Lorazepam (Ativan), given either by mouth or by intramuscular injection enjoys some popularity. This drug, as distinct from the other benzodiazepines, has a strong propensity to produce amnesia. The patient may not only be unaware of having been taken to the operating room but may also be unable to recollect the first few hours of the postoperative period. There is division of opinion as to whether this type of effect is to be desired, some patients being almost resentful of the fact that they cannot account for a significant part of the day in spite of the fact that they know that they were not anaesthetised for all of that time.

The phenothiazines. These drugs have been used to allay preoperative anxiety but their use has decreased in favour of the benzodiazepines. Many of the drugs in this group have important anti-emetic properties. The phenothiazines have few if any analgesic properties but they may be useful when combined with a small dose of an analgesic. A popular combination is a mixture of pethidine with promethazine in children. Trimeprazine (Vallergan) syrup is a palatable preparation and is widely used.

Droperidol belongs to a group of compounds known as the butyrophenones. It is sometimes used to supplement the sedative effects of the opiates and it has an anti-emetic effect. It is capable of producing an unpleasant feeling of dissociation in the patient, however, and its popularity in premedication is decreasing.

Postoperative vomiting. This can occur for many reasons. Sometimes it is a consequence of drugs which have been given for premedication, analgesia or postoperative pain relief. Sometimes it is associated with the operation or the disease necessitating the operating and sometimes it would seem to be almost self-induced by the patient who may expect to be sick after an anaesthetic and operation. While it would be foolish to claim that no one should vomit or feel nauseated in the postoperative period, reassurance and the appropriate drugs can reduce the frequency of postoperative vomiting and nausea to the point at which a patient might normally expect to be free from these unpleasant symptoms. Drugs used normally as premedicants such as hyoscine and the phenothiazines may reduce the frequency of vomiting. Specific anti-emetic therapy would involve the use of such drugs as cyclizine and metoclopramide (Maxolon). The combination of cyclizine with morphine (Cyclimorph) is a fashionable commercial preparation. The phenothiazine group of compounds gives a wide choice but promazine (Sparine), although perhaps less fashionable these days, is very effective.

Oral premedication. Several of the drugs mentioned above, notably the benzodiazepines, may be given orally. While this route of administration may seem to be a contradiction in view of the need for fasting before anaesthesia, it is generally accepted that there will be little risk of regurgitation as a consequence of taking a small sip of water. Oral premedication has many advantages over injection. Not only do patients prefer premedication in which the unpleasantness of a needle is avoided but the work of the nursing staff is much reduced also. Oral premedication has obvious advantages in the preparation of children for surgery and helps to maintain the trust that the nursing and medical team may have established with the patient.

The nurse should be aware of the need to observe patients who have received premedicant drugs while ensuring that they are allowed to benefit from the drugs in tranquil surroundings. As a rule the anaesthetist will depend on the nursing staff to ensure that the premedication has been given at the agreed time. If for any reason the drugs have not been given at that time it is essential that the anaesthetist should be advised of this and it must not be assumed that late administration is better than none at all. Not only might the patient gain no benefit from the sedatives incorporated in a premedicant prescription, but the drugs may exert their maximum depressant activity during anaesthesia when depression from other drugs is already maximal.

Neuroleptanalgesia
Local analgesia
Regional blocks

Induced (controlled)
   hypotension
Endotracheal anaesthesia

6

Some special techniques

NEUROLEPTANALGESIA

Certain minor neurosurgical procedures and diagnostic procedures, such as cardiac catheterisation, may ideally be performed in patients who are sedated and free from pain, where muscular relaxation is not essential. The patient's co-operation is occasionally required during the procedure and therefore he or she should be capable of being aroused. This stage of sedation and indifference to environment, combined with analgesia and the ability to co-operate when required, is known as neuroleptanalgesia. As yet, no one drug can produce these conditions, but various combinations have been tried with more or less success.

The drugs used in this technique comprise:

Neuroleptic drugs which produce a state of dissociation—usually a pleasant sensation but sometimes associated with acute anxiety. The best known is dehydrobenzperidol (Droperidol) which is a potent anti-emetic agent and is claimed to protect the circulation against the 'shock' of surgery. Unfortunately, it may also cause Parkinsonian tremors and delayed feelings of disorientation.

Potent analgesics—fentanyl and phenoperidine. Fentanyl (Sublimaze) is related chemically to pethidine and 0.1 mg is approximately equipotent with morphine 10 mg. The duration of analgesia with fentanyl is about 20–40 minutes. It shares with pethidine the ability to produce nausea and vomiting, cardiorespiratory depression and, in the long term, addiction. Phenoperidine (Operidine) has pharmacological effects very similar to those of fentanyl except that the duration of analgesia of 2 mg of the drug (= 10 mg of morphine) is about 90 minutes.

Mixtures of fentanyl with droperidol (Thalamonal) may be used to induce a state of unconsciousness with profound analgesia. Anaesthesia is maintained, thereafter, with nitrous oxide and oxygen and, when required, a muscle relaxant drug (see also p. 18). While it is claimed that a stable arterial pressure and some protection from shock is provided by the neuroleptanalgesic combination of drugs, it is the opinion of many that, apart from the duration of action of fentanyl and phenoperidine, the advantage of neuroleptanalgesia over the use of the more traditional analgesics such as morphine in the maintenance of anaesthesia is not striking.

LOCAL ANALGESIA

All patients who are to be operated on under some form of local or regional analgesia should receive the same care and attention as other patients undergoing surgery. They should be starved and premedicated for all but the most minor procedures. This enables a general anaesthetic to be given if necessary during the operation. The site of injection should be cleaned, if necessary shaved, and clothing loosened so as to make the area accessible when required.

The patient should be given a clear explanation of what is to be done and reassured that it is not an unpleasant experience. If some sedation is to be given together with the local analgesic it is important that the patient should not become confused or drowsy. For many types of local anaesthetic procedures the patient's co-operation is necessary to ensure proper positioning and it is best to give a preliminary account of what is required so that requests made in the anaesthetic room or operating theatre, when the patient's anxiety may be heightened, are reasonably familiar.

Equipment for local or regional analgesia

In many hospitals much of the equipment used is made up in disposable packs supplemented as necessary with ampoules of drugs, needles and cannulae. The anaesthetist will require towel, gown and gloves, swabs and a container for cleaning fluid used in preparing the skin, syringes and needles of various sizes, including, when required, special needles such as spinal needles and extradural (Tuohy type) needles, and an epidural catheter. This may be packed as a basic set supplemented for each technique, or individual sets may be pre-set depending on the local requirements. Disposable packs are widely available (see p. 40).

REGIONAL BLOCKS

Digital nerve block (finger or toe)

This is the simplest block (excluding local infiltration). After the hand is cleaned local analgesic is injected (*without* adrenaline) in a ring round the base of a digit. After a few minutes the digit is analgesic and ready for surgery.

Brachial plexus block

With the patient lying on his back the arm is extended and rotated outwards with the elbow flexed, the hand being supported by an assistant. The axilla is cleaned and towelled and local analgesic is injected on either side of the axillary artery.

Alternatively, with the patient lying on his back, the side to be blocked is prepared by an assistant pulling the hand down close by the side. The head is turned to face the other side and the supraclavicular area cleaned and towelled. Local analgesic is placed in the area of the first rib by injecting above the mid-point of the clavicle, the needle being directed inwards, backwards and downwards.

It is essential to give these and all local injections ample time to work.

Intravenous local analgesia (Bier's block)

This can be used for upper or lower limb surgery but in practice it is used more commonly to facilitate surgery in the arm.

A specially designed double cuff (Fig. 6.1) is placed around the patient's arm and connected to a sphygmomanometer column. The systolic arterial pressure is recorded. A needle or disposable plastic cannula is introduced to a vein away from the site of injury. The

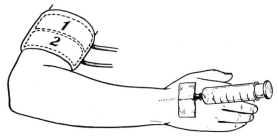

Figure 6.1 Intravenous local analgesia. The upper cuff is inflated after the limb has been rendered bloodless. The injection is then made, the lower cuff inflated and finally the upper one deflated.

limb is raised and emptied of blood with an Esmarch bandage. The upper cuff is then inflated to a pressure greater than the systolic arterial pressure, the Esmarch bandage removed and the local analgesic solution injected through the needle or cannula. For a 70 kg adult 40 ml of lignocaine 0.5% without adrenaline is used in the arm and as much as 100 ml in the leg.

The lower cuff is now inflated to a pressure greater than the systolic pressure and the upper cuff released. In this way the inflated cuff presses only on analgesic tissue.

The analgesic solution becomes fixed in the tissues in about 20 minutes after injection and is then slowly released and broken down in the body. If the operation lasts for a shorter time the cuff must be released carefully and reinflated to allow the solution to pass slowly into the general circulation. In this way side-effects are minimised.

Spinal (subarachnoid) and epidural (extradural) block

The advantages and disadvantages of these two methods are discussed in Chapter 3. It must again be stressed that in preparing for either of these two techniques absolute sterility must be observed. The towels, swabs, drugs, needles and syringes and any other instruments used by the anaesthetist, such as special adaptors, are best presented as a special pack which has been autoclaved. This procedure can be simplified if presterilised, disposable syringes and catheters (Fig. 6.2) are used. Where these are available it is necessary to keep only separate autoclaved supplies of the local analgesic solutions and needles to meet the preferences of individual anaesthetists. Before embarking on either of these techniques

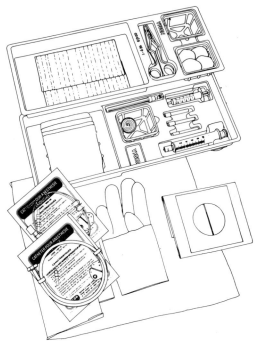

Figure 6.2 Disposable epidural (extradural) pack comprising needle with movable wings and a catheter.

secure access to a vein should be assured by inserting a cannula and fixing it carefully in position.

In preparing the skin the same care should be exercised as before a laparotomy. The staff concerned should wear cap, mask, gloves and gown.

After a pack containing autoclaved ampoules has been opened any unused ampoules should be discarded and replaced. Repeated autoclaving may reduce the potency of the drugs.

The drugs used are essentially those used for local analgesia.

Local analgesic solutions

Strength of solution

The local analgesic drugs act on the nerve fibre to block conduction. The thin sympathetic fibres are blocked by dilute solutions, the medium sized sensory (pain carrying) fibres by stronger solutions, and the motor fibres, which control movement, by still stronger solutions. Recovery takes place in reverse order, the patient being able to move before he feels pain, and feel pain while his blood vessels are dilated.

Use of adrenaline. Adrenaline is added to local analgesic solutions because it causes the blood vessels to contract. By so doing it slows the absorption of the local analgesic into the blood stream. Consequently, the local action is prolonged and, as less is absorbed in a given period of time, toxic effects are not so likely. However, as the blood vessels are constricted, adrenaline must never be used in the area of vessels supplying a part which has no other blood supply, such as the finger or penis lest the tissue receive insufficient oxygen to keep it alive and gangrene results. Figure 6.3 shows what happened when a local analgesic solution, containing adrenaline, was injected at the base of a septic thumb.

The information required in preparing an injection of a local analgesic solution consists of the following:

What drug is being used?

How much is required either in millilitres or milligrams? It is useful to remember that 1 ml of a 1% solution contains 10 mg.

Is adrenaline required and in what strength? A concentration of 1 : 300 000 is adequate for the effects noted above and greater concentrations should not be used.

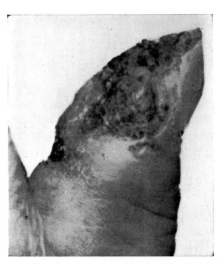

Figure 6.3 Gangrene resulting from injection of local analgesic solution containing adrenaline at the base of the thumb.

All this information should be obtained from the anaesthetist and checked on the bottle or ampoule and re-checked by another nurse. The drugs for injection must always be drawn from the labelled bottle or ampoule by the doctor giving the injection. The old practice of presenting solutions for injection in unlabelled containers is to be deprecated since accidents, such as mistaken injection of a sterilising fluid, can occur.

Remember that local analgesic drugs given in overdose (unnecessarily large volume or concentration or both) are as dangerous as any general anaesthetic given in overdose.

INDUCED (CONTROLLED) HYPOTENSION

It is sometimes an advantage to the surgeon to have the patient's arterial pressure at a level lower than normal. This reduces the bleeding at the site of operation and may make the dissection of tissues easier. This technique may be of value in the following circumstances.

When considerable blood loss is anticipated, for example abdomino-perineal resection of rectum.

When even a drop of blood may obscure the site of operation, for example operations in the ear performed with the aid of a microscope.

Hypotension is achieved by causing the blood vessels to dilate and by posturing the patient so that the blood pools in the lower parts of the body, away from the site of operation.

Most of the drugs used paralyse part of the sympathetic nervous system controlling blood vessels thus causing vasodilation. Some drugs have a direct relaxing effect on the muscles within blood vessels. The drugs include trimetaphan (Arfonad), and sodium nitroprusside which are given by intravenous injection. A similar result can be obtained by spinal or epidural block with a local anaesthetic. The arterial pressure may also be lowered by ventilating a patient with halothane where muscular relaxation has been achieved by giving curare.

While in some cases the blood pressure will have been allowed to return to normal or assisted to do so before the patient leaves the operating theatre, it is important that these patients are not allowed to sit up for some time or severe hypotension may return. Clear *written* instructions as to the management of each patient should be obtained from the anaesthetist to ensure correct supervision of the patient during the postoperative period.

ENDOTRACHEAL ANAESTHESIA

Administration of anaesthetic gases through an endotracheal tube is a widely used method for these reasons:

It allows the surgeon easier access to the face, head and neck during anaesthesia and permits maintenance of a clear airway under difficult circumstances, for example when the patient is lying face down.

It facilitates artificial ventilation, by ensuring that the gases are delivered to the lungs only and do not distend the stomach as positive pressure is applied. The use of a cuffed tube ensures a gas tight fit in the trachea.

A cuffed tube minimises the risk of inhalation of gastric contents in patients liable to vomit or regurgitate, and prevents the inhalation of blood in operations on the mouth, throat or nose.

The tubes used may be made of synthetic material such as polyvinyl chloride or of natural rubber (Fig. 6.4). They may be 'plain' or have an inflatable cuff attached to them (Fig. 6.5). In addition, the uncuffed tubes may be intended for insertion through

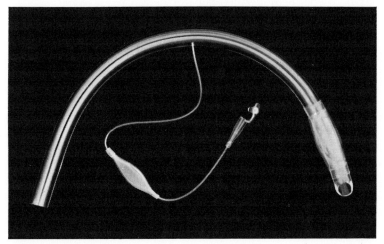

Figure 6.4 A cuffed 'Portex' tube. This tube is disposable.

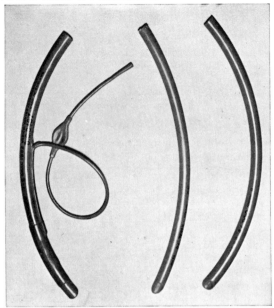

Figure 6.5 Three types of rubber endotracheal tubes in common use: from above down, plain-oral and nasal tubes and a cuffed oral tube.

the mouth, these being marked 'oral'. Others are intended for passage through the nose and these tubes are of thinner material and are clearly marked 'nasal'.

Latex tubes, reinforced by coils of nylon embedded in the wall, may be used where the tube is particularly likely to kink.

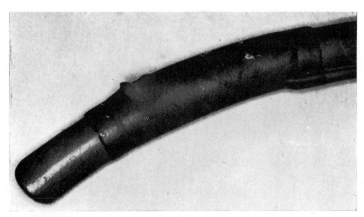

Figure 6.6 This figure shows an endotracheal tube with a defective cuff. A small area of the cuff has been weakened by repeated autoclaving.

After use, rubber tubes are carefully washed with water or approved solution and thoroughly cleaned both inside and out. The inside should be cleaned only with a brush and under no circumstances should a pledget of wool be pushed through instead. Thereafter the cuff should be tested by inflating it with a few millilitres of air. On inflation, the cuff should distend evenly with air. If a bubble appears on one or other side of the cuff, the tube should be condemned as this may cause the bevel of the tube to jam against the side of the trachea, thus obstructing the airway (Figs. 6.6 and 6.7). When the tube has been cleaned and tested it should be sterilised, preferably by high vacuum autoclaving. Most tubes will withstand this treatment about six times, but if they appear to kink easily or to show signs of cuff weakness they should be discarded or submitted to the anaesthetist for his opinion on their fitness for further service. The use of endotracheal tubes which show signs of wear and tear is a dangerous economy.

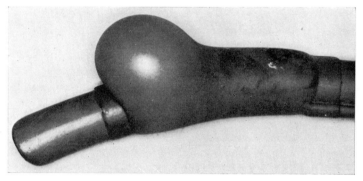

Figure 6.7 The same tube as in Figure 6.6 with the cuff partly inflated demonstrates the weak portion of the cuff which could result in displacement of the tube and respiratory obstruction.

In and around
theatre

Transport to the anaesthetic room

When taking or escorting a patient from the ward to the anaesthetic room, nursing and other staff all have a duty to ensure that the patient does not suffer any injury. Many patients will be drowsy but even the patient who is wide awake cannot see where he or she is going when lying on a trolley. Arms are most liable to be damaged: either an elbow protruding from the side of the trolley may strike a door or wall causing a fracture, or the arm, projecting, may catch on a door causing dislocation of the shoulder (Fig. 7.1). It is usually necessary for two people to undertake the transport of a patient and at least one of them should be a nurse.

In the anaesthetic room

On arrival in the anaesthetic room the patient should be treated in one of two ways. The sleeping patient should not be disturbed but positioned so that injury to limbs or nerves is avoided (Fig. 7.2). The awake patient should be engaged in reassuring conversation— perhaps with a simple explanation of the function of the apparatus and equipment in the anaesthetic room. Never carry on a conversation with others present unless you include the patient and do not discuss other patients. Just before induction of anaesthesia ensure

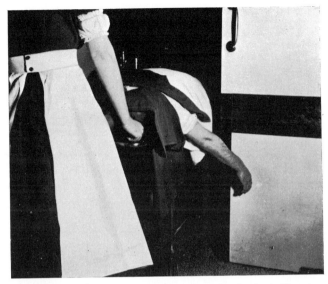

Figure 7.1 Failure to secure the patient's arm as the patient is wheeled into theatre may result in injury to the arm or shoulder.

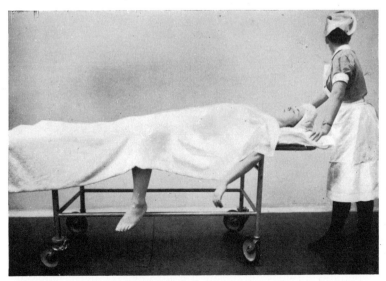

Figure 7.2 Inattention on the part of the nurse may result in the patient's limbs hanging from the trolley with possible damage to the nerves. The use of the type of trolley illustrated in Figure 7.27 obviates this type of injury.

that the patient is fully prepared for the operation to be carried out. The theatre gown should either be loosened at the neck or removed completely as for chest surgery. A diathermy plate covered with a saline pad may be attached to the leg at this stage or preferably when the patient is asleep but *not* during induction of anaesthesia.

Four golden rules for the anaesthetic room are:

Never leave a patient alone.

Do not allow a patient to sit up or get off the trolley unless there are at least two people to provide support.

Make yourself familiar with the whereabouts of essential equipment such as suction apparatus since you may require it in a hurry.

Maintain a calm and reassuring demeanour. During induction of anaesthesia hearing is the last of the senses to be lost and may be temporarily exaggerated; in this state the patient may mistake the clatter of a metal basin for the apocalypse!

No attempt is made here to list the contents of the anaesthetic room, or the setting up of the apparatus or drugs before a surgical session begins. This is a matter for instruction on the spot by the sister or anaesthetist as the variations in individual requirements and available facilities are almost limitless.

THE NURSE AS ASSISTANT IN THE ADMINISTRATION OF ANAESTHESIA

Intravenous induction

Where the intravenous route is to be used to induce anaesthesia a suitable vein should be exposed, normally on the back of the patient's hand (Fig. 7.3). This site is preferable as it is less likely that the needle will enter an artery in error, or that a nerve will be damaged. An alternative site, although never preferred to the back of the hand, is the antecubital fossa. When the chosen vein is exposed, the nurse should compress the arm above the area intended for injection, leaving plenty of room for access to the vein. After the anaesthetist has punctured the vein, usually with a disposable needle or cannula (Figs. 7.4 and 7.5), he will indicate when the nurse should release the pressure. The nurse should not allow the arm to drop, and adequate support should be given until all the injections have been completed and the cannula is secured

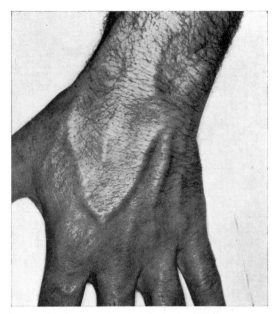

Figure 7.3 The superficial venous plexus on the back of the hand is a suitable site for drug injection.

in position with adhesive tape. Such support is particularly important after the patient has lost consciousness. After the needle has been withdrawn from the vein, particularly if the injection has been made on the dorsum of the hand, a firm pad such as a piece of

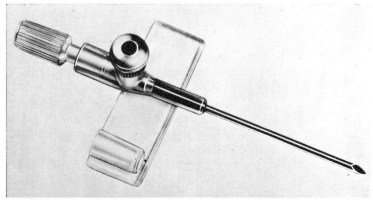

Figure 7.4 The Viggo Needle. Injections may be made through the rubber diaphragm on the top of the needle. The plastic plug in the hub of the needle may be removed and injections or infusions delivered by this route.

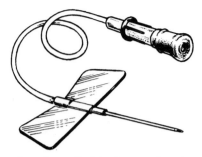

Figure 7.5 The Abbott Butterfly needle. Injections are given through the rubber diaphragm attached to the needle by a plastic tube.

dental roll should be firmly placed over the site of injection to prevent a troublesome haematoma developing. The arm should then be secured at the side or in the patient's gown. Under no circumstances should the hand be tucked under the buttock or severe damage by pressure may result.

Inhalation induction

The procedure in this case is quite different. The induction will last longer and may be accompanied by some struggling as the patient passes through the stage of excitement. To many patients it is a great comfort to hold the hand of the nurse they have known in the ward as they go off to sleep. It is better that the nurse should hold the patient's hand and in such a way that her own cannot be crushed (Fig. 7.6).

If the patient should move or struggle, it is very important that restraint should only be applied if he is liable to damage himself or others, or if the induction is likely to be interrupted. Even then, only minimal force should be used (Fig. 7.7) otherwise a violent struggle may ensue, and with an uninhibited patient the outcome is sometimes in doubt! During inhalation induction the patient loses consciousness slowly, the last sense to be lost being that of hearing. Long after the patient is apparently asleep remarks about him or his condition should be avoided. Comments about other patients should not be made lest the patient interpret them as applying to himself.

In the case of children it may be particularly distressing to the patient and the onlookers if induction is not smooth. When the child is asleep after premedication it may be possible to waft an

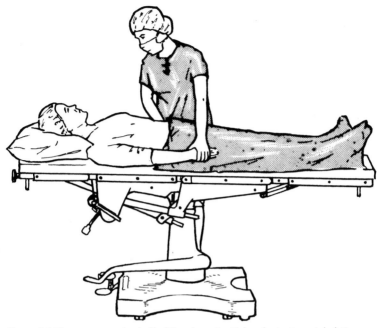

Figure 7.6 The correct method of holding the patient's hand prior to an inhalation induction of anaesthesia.

inhalation anaesthetic mixture over the nose as an effective prelude to applying a mask. The rational child may be persuaded to breathe from a mask as if it were part of a game. Where possible many anaesthetists offer the child a choice of injection or breathing from a mask. If a child resists all efforts at obtaining co-operation the quickest, least traumatic, method is the safest but whatever is done will seem relatively inelegant.

After induction of anaesthesia a tracheal tube (Ch. 6) may be inserted and the nurse can help in this manoeuvre by retracting the lip at the right hand corner of the patient's mouth, thus improving the anaesthetist's field of vision (Fig. 7.8). The nurse should also be available to pass tubes or packs to the anaesthetist when required.

If spinal, epidural or local analgesia is to be used, the anaesthetist will normally indicate the desired position of the patient and the nurse may be expected to help to achieve and maintain this position. It is probably better to be silent during the induction of this form of analgesia so that the patient's attention is not distracted from any instructions given by the anaesthetist.

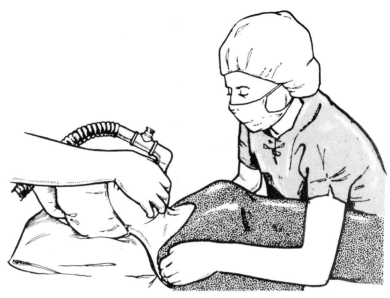

Figure 7.7 The nurse is assisting the anaesthetist by restraining the patient while allowing free movement of the chest and abdomen.

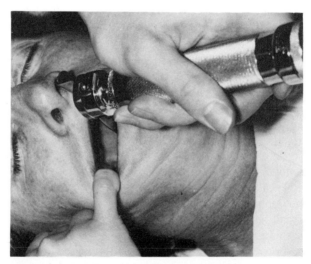

Figure 7.8 A finger retracting the patient's lip during laryngoscopy greatly increases the anaesthetist's field of vision.

Induction of anaesthesia in a patient who may have a full stomach may require the further co-operation of the nurse. In addition to the precautions described previously (p. 23) anaesthesia may be induced with the patient tilted into a head-up position to lessen the risk of regurgitation, or in the head down position or lateral head down position to lessen the risk of flow of gastric contents into the bronchial tree. The patient may be placed head-up position initially in the knowledge that the table or trolley can be placed in the head-down position very rapidly if regurgitation ensues. This may be done on the operating table or on a special tilting trolley. Pressure on the cricoid cartilage (Fig. 7.9) during induction obstructs the oesophagus and prevents regurgitation of stomach contents and the nurse should be experienced in performing this manoeuvre.

Transport from the anaesthetic room to the operating table

All parts of the patient's body, particularly joints must be protected against injury and everyone present should ensure that the infusion, anaesthetic and other types of tubing and connection are not disrupted.

In theatre

The patient should be placed on to the operating table in the appropriate position for the operation to be carried out (Figs. 7.10–7.16). One arm will normally be placed on a support and be used

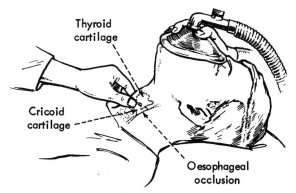

Figure 7.9 Firm pressure on the cricoid by an assistant during induction of anaesthesia may prevent regurgitation of stomach contents by occluding the oesophagous.

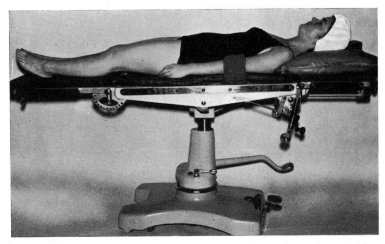

Figure 7.10 The supine position used for the majority of surgical procedures. In this and subsequent positions where the patient is lying on her back some form of support is placed under the ankles to avoid pressure on the calves. This pressure increases the risk of venous stasis and thrombosis. A lumbar support would also be used.

for infusion and injections. If there is no contraindication, it is usual to use the arm on the side away from that at which the surgeon will be operating. Arterial pressure monitoring (arm cuff), e.c.g. and other monitoring arrangements should be set up and operating fully

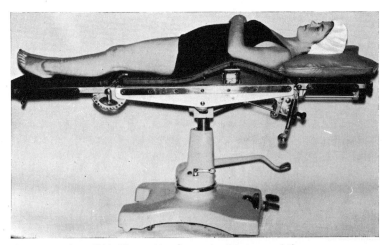

Figure 7.11 The gall-bladder position: in practice the arm would be on an arm-board.

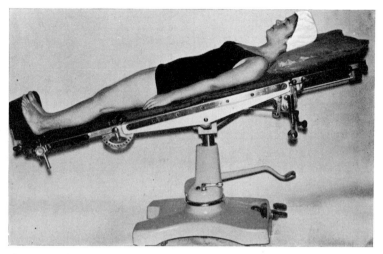

Figure 7.12 The reversed Trendelenburg position: if a non-slip mattress is not used then the foot-rest shown here is essential.

before the sterile drapes, which obscure the patient to a variable extent, are applied.

The correct position for an arm board is shown in Figure 7.17. Note that the arm should not be below the level of the body or more than a right angle from the side.

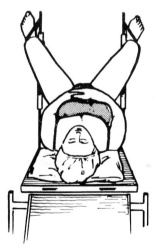

Figure 7.13 The lithotomy position: although other types of stirrups or leg supports can be used, care must always be taken to prevent undue pressure on the blood vessels and nerves of the leg.

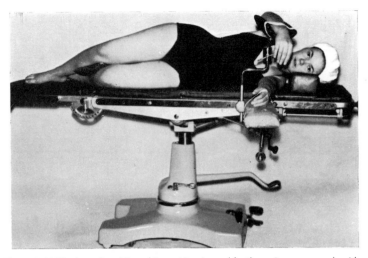

Figure 7.14 The lateral position: this position is used for thoracic surgery and, with the table broken, gives good exposure for operations on the kidney. Note the pad inserted between the legs. As in all other positions great care must be taken that no contact is made between the patient and bare metal on the table or its supports.

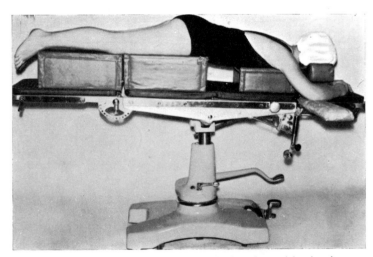

Figure 7.15 The prone position: the blocks support the pelvis and the chest but permit free movement of the abdominal wall during respiration. The slight head-down tilt improves bronchial drainage during operation.

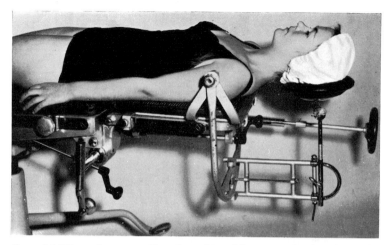

Figure 7.16 The endoscopy position: the position of the patient's head can be altered to facilitate examination during bronchoscopy or oesophagoscopy.

Measurement of blood loss

Where considerable blood loss is anticipated it is important to measure blood loss and replace blood promptly (Figs. 7.18 and 7.19) and with a filter if necessary (Fig. 7.20). The anaesthetist obtains information about the state of the circulation by recording the arterial blood pressure and the heart rate regularly. In some

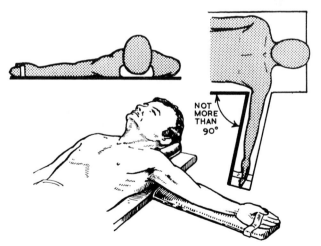

Figure 7.17 The correct position of the arm-board as shown.

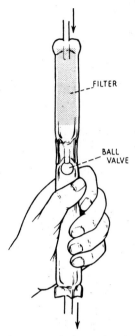

Figure 7.18 A pressure transfusion set. The lower chamber is allowed to fill with blood and when the full chamber is again compressed the ball occludes the upper outlet and blood is forced down the tubing to the patient.

cases the central venous pressure may be measured using a simple manometer. The nurse may assist, however, by weighing used swabs, measuring the blood in suction bottles and by estimating other sources of blood loss as on towels and the operating table or floor. In some circumstances in which blood loss must be known accurately all towels or swabs are washed in a special machine and the washings analysed photoelectrically to determine the blood loss. Although swab weighing may be less accurate than the photoelectric methods it gives a good indication of blood loss (Fig. 7.21).

Temperature of blood

Blood stored in a refrigerator will be transfused at a temperature below that of the body—the difference varying with the time lapse between removal and transfusion and the rate of transfusion. With slow transfusions of relatively small amounts of blood the lower

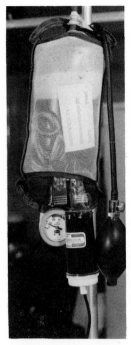

Figure 7.19 Device for the administration of blood to a vein under pressure. The bag containing blood is enclosed in a cuff which is inflated by squeezing the bulb. The pressure gauge is designed to show the maximum safe pressure which can be used.

temperature of the blood is of little consequence. Where, however, large quantities of cold blood are transfused rapidly, a severe fall in body temperature may result leading to a cardiac arrest. Steps must therefore be taken to warm the blood to body temperature. This may be done by warming the bottle or container or by passing the blood through a coil immersed in warm water en route to the patient (Fig. 7.22).

When massive blood transfusions are given there will be concern that the patient's blood chemistry and coagulation mechanisms are not impaired and the help of the appropriate laboratories will be needed.

Transfer of the patient

Transferring the patient from the trolley to the table and back to the trolley at the end of operation is a matter which is now deservedly

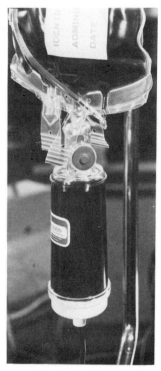

Figure 7.20 Blood filter.

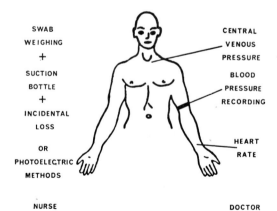

Figure 7.21 Methods of assessing blood loss. The methods in which the nurse assists are shown on the left of the diagram.

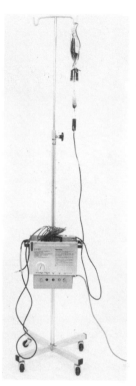

Figure 7.22 Blood warmer.

receiving considerable attention. For many years this was achieved by lifting the patient on a stretcher with poles. In view of the variation in height between trolleys, tables and beds this can be a very awkward manoeuvre and has doubtless contributed to the high incidence of backache in personnel faced with this problem. There are a number of alternatives. One is to ensure that when a patient is lifted there are sufficient staff available to ensure that this does not impose too great a burden on any individual. Alternatively, the use of suitable rollers (Fig. 7.23) allows the patient to be rolled rather than lifted from table to trolley. A rubber sheet rolls over a number of fixed rollers and the roller and patient travel together in the same direction. While this still involves handling the patient the effort involved is considerably reduced. Another solution to this problem is the use of special trolleys, the tops of which are detachable and clamp to a pedestal in the theatre forming the top of the operating table.

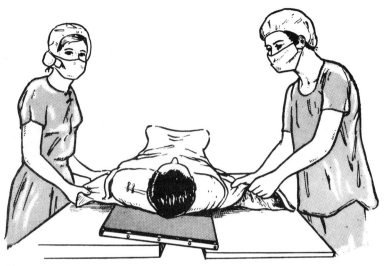

Figure 7.23 A patient roller in use.

A further problem associated with transport of patients is that of their transfer to and from the sterile operating suite. Special trolleys (Fig. 7.24) have been designed with tops which slide from one base outside the sterile area to another inside the area.

Returning the patient to the ward

During the operation itself the ward nurse, if present in theatre, acts as a link with the ward and will observe intelligently what is taking place so that she or he can report later to the ward sister. At the end of the operation steps should be taken to ensure that intravenous infusions are properly secured for transport to the ward. When a

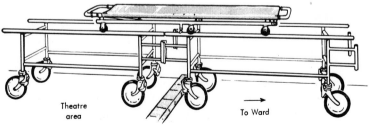

Theatre
area

To Ward

Figure 7.24 The Thackray transfer trolley system.

cannula has been used, minimal splintage will be required. In other cases the splint should be applied to immobilise the limb in such a way that the needle is not displaced. If a water-seal drain has been inserted into the chest, after thoracic operation, it should be adequately clamped (using *two* clamps) before moving the patient to the trolley. Transfer of the patient to the trolley should be carried out with great care, as it is possible, at this stage, to cause a severe reduction in arterial pressure by rough handling.

Before leaving theatre with the patient for the journey back to the recovery room make sure that:

The anaesthetist considers the patient fit to leave theatre. It sometimes happens that a patient may not be breathing adequately and the anaesthetist may wish to observe the response to treatment either in theatre or in the recovery room.

There are instructions for the after-care of the patient. This information—what sedation is to be given and what infusions have to be continued—should always be clearly written on a special instruction sheet.

There is adequate assistance for the journey. At least two people are required to transport an unconscious patient, and the nurse or doctor should be at the patient's head. It is usually necessary to support the patient's chin to ensure a clear airway (Figs. 7.25 and

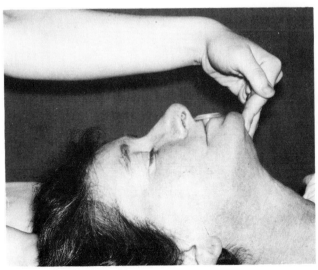

Figure 7.25

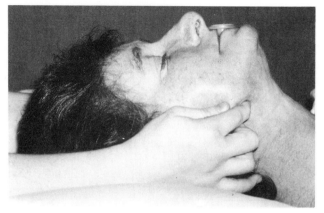

Figure 7.26

7.26). The use of a tilting trolley with sides (Fig. 7.27) ensures greater safety on the journey back to the recovery room or ward. The patient lies on her or his side in a slightly head down position. Oxygen may be administered if required and gags, laryngoscope, portable suction and other apparatus are available on a tray below the trolley. Such a trolley may serve the patient as a bed throughout the recovery period.

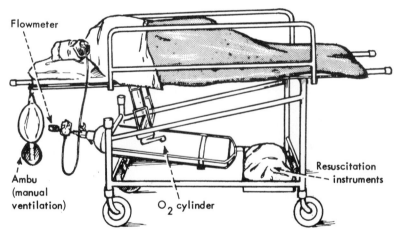

Flowmeter

Ambu
(manual
ventilation)

O_2 cylinder

Resuscitation
instruments

Figure 7.27 Patient on tilting trolley awaiting transfer to the recovery room. The cylinder of oxygen lies below the trolley and the mechanism for tilting is above the cylinder.

Despite a long standing and mainly traditional objection, it is much better to return a patient feet first to the recovery room or ward, as the nurse at the head has better control of the chin, can observe the patient and can see where she is going. The person at the foot of the trolley has little to do but help propel the trolley and can walk beside it, or indeed backwards, without endangering the patient.

8

In and around the labour room

Much of what is said throughout this book applies to all patients about to receive an anaesthetic and the general principles described apply equally to obstetric patients. There are, however, some additional problems encountered in patients in labour and some of these are considered further in this section.

The full stomach

Where elective procedures such as elective Caesarean section or external version are contemplated preparation of the patient is similar to that for any other planned operation (p. 23).

Many patients, however, undergo operative obstetric procedures at the end of a varying period of labour and during labour gastric emptying may be considerably delayed. It is clearly impracticable to starve every patient in labour because only a few may require a general anaesthetic and, as this would lead to severe acidosis in many cases, such starvation would be frankly dangerous. Many centres, however, now restrict the feeding of patients in labour to a liquid diet and recourse may be had to intravenous fluids as a supplement or alternative. This ensures that the stomach may be more easily emptied by tube if necessary and lessens the hazard of vomiting or regurgitation. The routine administration of antacids at

2 to 3 hourly intervals during labour will also ensure that the stomach contents remain alkaline.

When considering the problem of emptying the stomach of a patient in labour the presence of the unborn baby and placenta may force one to abandon the use of oesophageal or stomach tubes. The passage of such a tube is often associated with retching, coughing and straining which may cause transient hypoxia in the mother and thus the baby or, in a patient who has had an ante-partum haemorrhage, may result in further massive bleeding. In such cases antacid therapy (see p. 24) is used and the anaesthetist will use other means including cricoid pressure during induction of anaesthesia to prevent aspiration of stomach content into the lungs (p. 53).

Premedication for general anaesthesia for obstetric procedures

As most, if not all, sedative drugs used for normal premedication pass the placental barrier into the fetus it is normal practice to omit sedatives from the premedication and to administer atropine alone. As many obstetric operations are carried out at very short notice there is much to be said for giving this drug intravenously. Increasingly with the use of ultra-light anaesthesia for obstetric operations, complaints of awareness during operation have been made by patients. An attempt to reduce this may be made by giving hyoscine or diazepam as premedication. More recently, low concentrations of halothane have been given during the anaesthetic to overcome this problem.

Provision of analgesia during labour

Labour is divided into three stages, the first stage up to full dilatation of the cervix, the second from then until the child is delivered, the third till the placenta is delivered.

During the early stage of labour, when the contractions of the uterus are felt as discomfort rather than pain, it is traditional to use mild sedatives to control this discomfort. In some patients where anxiety is present the use of small doses of a 'tranquilliser' or barbiturate may be tried. It is, however, essential to remember that when using a barbiturate in the presence of pain in such cases, excitement and restlessness may be produced.

The regular severe contractions, felt as definite and increasing pains, are usually controlled by the administration of a more potent analgesic drug. The one most favoured is pethidine, given in doses of 100 mg intramuscularly. Morphine, which is an effective analgesic and provides some degree of sedation also, has fallen from favour because of the respiratory depression which it may cause and the likelihood that this might interfere with the start of respiration of the child. It is now believed that the degree of respiratory depression produced by pethidine is almost as great as that produced by morphine, in the equivalent dosage. Pethidine is, however, claimed to facilitate dilatation of the cervix during labour and its lack of sedative properties and production of respiratory depression have been overcome in two ways.

To enhance its sedative properties it may be given with a phenothiazine drug, such as promazine, and this combination has been used with apparently favourable results by some obstetricians. To overcome the respiratory depression which it causes, pethidine has been mixed with the antagonist drug levallorphan. The value of this combination is questioned by some and, if an antagonist drug is required, it may be better to administer it separately either to the patient or to the child after delivery. Nalorphine (Lethidrone) or levallorphan may be used for this purpose. The use of uterine paracervical block for relief of pain late in the first stage of labour has much to recommend it since depression of the fetus is avoided.

The objections to the use of the non-volatile sedative or analgesic agents, because they produce depression of the fetus, can be minimised by restricting their use to the early part of labour, that is before the cervix is fully dilated. From then on until the child is delivered it is customary to use volatile or gaseous analgesic agents, which are rapidly excreted by the mother and should cause minimal fetal depression. The two possibilities are that nitrous oxide in oxygen is inhaled or that low concentrations of trichloroethylene or methoxyflurane in air are used. In this country, midwives may administer nitrous oxide with 50% oxygen, trichloroethylene or methoxyflurane from specially designed inhalers.

Nitrous oxide and air air mixtures are not without hazard as the air comprises 50% of the mixture which therefore contains only 10% oxygen. Such mixtures are therefore not suitable for patients suffering from anaemia, cardiac disease, respiratory disease or hypertension. The use of these gas and air mixtures is now virtually obsolete.

The use of the more rational *nitrous oxide 50%: oxygen 50% mixture* has now become widespread since it has been possible to combine nitrous oxide and oxygen premixed in one cylinder such that it will normally be delivered in the same proportions and supplied on demand. If the cylinder has been exposed to severe cold—and many cylinders are stored outside even in winter—the gases may separate and when the cylinder is almost empty lower proportions oxygen are supplied. This can be prevented by inverting the cylinders several time before use. A special demand valve is used with the cylinder and the complete Entonox unit is shown in use in Figure 8.1.

Trichloroethylene (Trilene) may be administered in 0.35 or 0.5% concentrations in air from temperature compensated vaporisers which ensure that the percentage of Trilene is constant under all circumstances and this is a considerable step forward in this technique. Methoxyflurane has been used in similar fashion with good results (Figs. 8.2 and 8.3).

The use of these volatile or gaseous analgesics, from the stage of dilatation of the cervix to delivery of the child, is facilitated by the

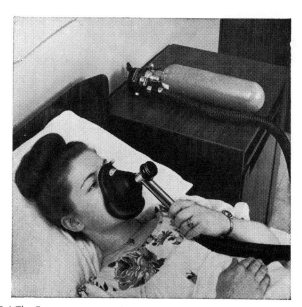

Figure 8.1 The Entonox apparatus in use.

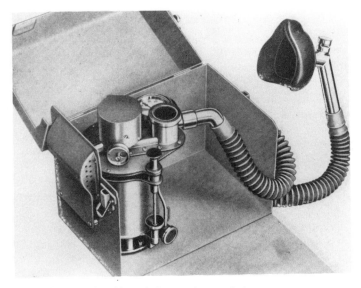

Figure 8.2 The Emotril trichloroethylene analgesia inhaler.

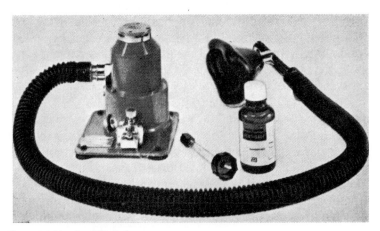

Figure 8.3 The Cardiff Inhaler.

previous administration of the non-volatile agents which have been described. This is particularly valuable where nitrous oxide and oxygen is to be administered as the hangover resulting from opiate or pethidine supplements the weak analgesic properties of these agents. The patient should have had some antenatal instruction in the use of the analgesic apparatus and should be told to take some deep breaths of the mixture with the onset of the first pain. Lack of antenatal instruction and inadequate supervision of the machines have tended to discredit this technique but, where properly used, it is valuable at this stage of labour.

Hypnosis and relaxation exercises

The teachings of Dr Grantly Dick Read regarding the value of relaxation during childbirth have been fairly widely accepted. Antenatal classes, where the patient is taught the technique of relaxation to be practised during the actual childbirth, are now common practice. This voluntary control and relaxation of specific muscle groups is undoubtedly of value and in many patients gives considerable relief from the pains of labour. Similarly some practitioners have found the use of hypnosis, when induced in the antenatal period and practised by the patient during labour, to be of considerable value. Hypnosis has undoubtedly some applications in this field—and some potential dangers—but when used by skilled hypnotists it undoubtedly produces good results in selected patients. It is not, however, generally considered to be an adequate substitute for other forms of analgesia.

Local and regional techniques

The danger of inhalation of stomach contents is clearly greatest during general anaesthesia and for this reason local analgesia is widely used for some obstetric procedures.

Local infiltration of the perineum can be used for the suture of perineal tears. Pudendal nerve block can be used for many low cavity forceps deliveries and paracervical uterine block is used by many obstetricians in the later stages of labour. Extradural analgesia is being used increasingly for operative work including Caesarean section. Low spinal anaesthesia is also becoming more popular again, particularly for forceps deliveries.

Resuscitation of the newborn

This tends to be the subject of considerable controversy and the practice varies from one hospital to another, not only as to who carries out the resuscitative measures but as to what measures are employed. In general, however, the resuscitation of the apnoeic infant follows the same principles that underlie the treatment of severe respiratory depression in any other circumstance. This involves clearing the airway of secretions by suction and administering oxygen, if necessary, by controlled ventilation often after endotracheal intubation.

Further reading

While we have outlined the principles of this important section of the treatment of the obstetric patient, for fuller details of the nursing preparation and techniques readers are referred to the appropriate chapters of the following:

Myles 1981   A textbook for midwives, 9th edn. Churchill Livingstone, Edinburgh

Moir D D 1982 Pain relief in labour, 4th edn. Churchill Livingstone, Edinburgh

9

Recovery room— after-care of patients

Ideally, all patients should be observed during the postoperative period in a centralised recovery room which is part of the operating theatre suite. The length of stay in such a room will depend on the condition of the patient and the nature of the surgical procedure and anaesthesia. Such an arrangement provides for the close observation of all patients during the crucial postoperative period, when consciousness and reflexes may still be impaired, and results in an economy of nursing and medical personnel and apparatus. In this country, however, some hospitals still do not have recovery facilities and some compromise is usually necessary. It should be possible, however, to nurse major surgical, seriously ill and emergency cases through the recovery period, in a side-ward near the theatre or in a screened section of a general ward. Whatever the local arrangement, it is essential that all nurses engaged in postoperative care should be trained specially for this work and be capable of carrying out certain emergency resuscitation manoeuvres.

COMPLICATIONS OF ANAESTHESIA

The complications requiring the special attention of the recovery room nursing staff readily fall into five groups:
1. Respiratory: obstruction of the airway; respiratory inadequacy and respiratory arrest.

73

2. Circulatory: hypotension; cardiac irregularities and cardiac arrest.
3. Gastro-intestinal; vomiting and regurgitation of stomach contents.
4. Renal.
5. Neurological sequelae.

These main groups overlap in many instances, e.g. a patient may regurgitate while still recovering from anaesthesia, inhale gastric contents and suffer respiratory obstruction. Untreated, this complication could lead to eventual cardiac arrest and death.

We will now consider these complications in more detail, describing their mechanism, their recognition and appropriate treatment.

Respiratory complications

Obstruction of the airway

The commonest respiratory complication, in the immediate postoperative period, is obstruction of the patient's upper airway. The three commonest causes are: the tongue falling back against the posterior wall of the pharynx when the patient is lying on his back; the presence of foreign material in the pharynx; and laryngeal spasm. Respiratory obstruction can usually be diagnosed when there are exaggerated movements of the chest and abdomen but very little air passes through the nose or mouth and the patient becomes increasingly cyanosed. Laryngeal spasm often results in a 'crowing' noise on inspiration as the air passes through the constricted larynx. An old axiom that is worth remembering here is that *noisy breathing is always obstructed breathing, but not all obstructed breathing is noisy.*

Treatment. Secure a clear airway immediately. This is usually readily accomplished by pulling the lower jaw upwards and forwards thus pulling the tongue away from the posterior pharyngeal wall. Only rarely should it be necessary to grip the tongue and pull it forward with forceps. Suction may be required to remove any foreign material causing obstruction, for example mucus. Oxygen may have to be administered but is quite useless unless the airway is already clear.

If no improvement follows these manoeuvres, *get help.*

Respiratory insufficiency

Despite an unobstructed upper airway, some patients, for one reason or another, may not breathe deeply enough to permit an adequate respiratory exchange to take place in the alveoli. Any interference with this mechanism results in hypoxia and carbon dioxide retention (Fig. 9.1). This may occur for many different reasons:

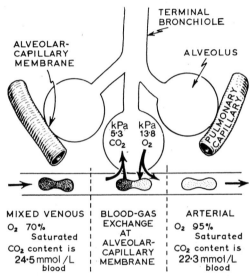

Figure 9.1 The alveolar-capillary diagram: this diagram demonstrates the blood-gas changes which take place during normal respiration as the blood passes through the lungs.

Obstruction of the smaller airways or bronchi.

Depression of the brain centres controlling respiration, following head injuries or cerebrovascular accidents, or the prolonged effects of anaesthetic agents.

Disease of or damage to the nervous pathways controlling the muscles of respiration, e.g. poliomyelitis.

Weakness of the muscles of respiration themselves as in myasthenia gravis, or when the action of muscle relaxant drugs has not been properly reversed at the end of the operation.

The operation itself, e.g. removal of lung tissue, as in lobectomy or pneumonectomy, may prevent adequate respiration.

Pre-existing lung disease may result in inadequate respiration, e.g. chronic bronchitis or emphysema.

Constriction of the chest wall or abdomen which interferes with normal expansion during breathing, can result in postoperative respiratory inadequacy. This may be the result of pre-existing disease of the thoracic cage, e.g. ankylosing spondylitis, or a simpler cause sometimes found in the application of too tight a dressing following operation.

Inadequate respiration may be recognised by the following signs:

Colour change. Cyanosis may be evident (hypoxia) or the skin may be red, hot and moist (carbon dioxide retention).

Respirations. These may be fast and shallow or abnormally slow. However, no matter what the respiratory rate or pattern, the other signs of respiratory inadequacy must never be ignored.

Pulse and blood pressure. In the early stages, the pulse is usually full, bounding and rapid, and the blood pressure rises. If the condition is allowed to persist then the pulse rate rises and the blood pressure falls.

Change in level of consciousness. If the patient has previously been conscious then respiratory inadequacy may be evidenced by increasing restlessness, confusion, drowsiness and eventual coma.

Treatment. Having secured a clear airway, the next step, no matter what the underlying cause of the respiratory inadequacy, must always be to assist the patient's own inadequate efforts. Increasing the amount of oxygen in the inspired air alone rarely results in improvement. Many simple devices are now available to augment the patient's ventilation. These enable the nurse or doctor to administer atmospheric air or oxygen by intermittent compression of a bag or bellows, e.g. Ambu resuscitator, Lucas bellows, etc (Fig. 9.2)

No properly equipped recovery room should be without one or other of these simple devices and all nursing staff should be skilled in their use. However, there may be circumstances when no apparatus is immediately available and the nurse must resort to other methods to support the patient's failing or absent ventilation. The simplest and most effective of these is the technique of expired air resuscitation or mouth to mouth breathing. A detailed description of this method is given in Chapter 11.

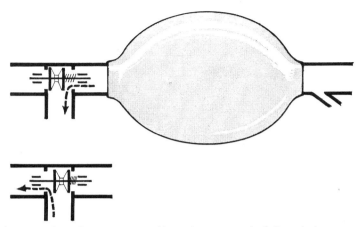

Figure 9.2 The Ambu resuscitator: additional oxygen may be fed into the bag through the small side tube at the right of the picture thus enriching the air which is driven into the patient's lungs when the bag is compressed. On the left of the illustration is the non-return valve connected to a mask or endotracheal tube by the vertical limb. The patient's expirations are delivered to the atmosphere through the horizontal limb of the valve.

Circulatory complications

When considering *circulatory changes* following anaesthesia, it is important to remember the significance of alterations in the patient's colour. Pallor, in the absence of other signs of shock, or flushing, in the absence of other signs of inadequate respiration, may be quite normal. Cyanosis *always* calls for rapid treatment.

The temperature of patients returning to a recovery room postoperatively may often be found to be slightly sub-normal. While it is important to prevent such patients shivering, only exceptionally should heat be applied, as this results in diversion of the blood from the vital organs to the skin.

Pulse

The pulse rate should be carefully observed during the immediate postoperative period.

A moderate tachycardia (80–100/min) commonly follows major surgery but a persistent tachycardia, particularly if it is increasing, should always be regarded as a danger sign, indicating perhaps haemorrhage or inadequate respiration.

Arterial pressure

Following a major operation the arterial pressure may be below the preoperative value, due to the effect of the surgery itself and the continuing action of drugs administered by the anaesthetist. A systolic arterial pressure of about 20 mm Hg (3 kPa) below the preoperative value can often be accepted, but where the blood pressure continues to fall or to rise unduly an explanation should be sought. All patients who have had a general anaesthetic, and some to whom a regional analgesic has been given, are particularly liable to hypotension and even sudden cardiac arrest if they are roughly handled or put in the sitting-up position (postural hypotension). All patients should be moved gently from trolley to bed and kept flat (or in the *tonsillar position*) until recovery is complete. In special cases, the bed may be tilted to a moderate head-down position for the first hour or two.

Frequent arterial pressure readings are time consuming and not usually necessary (e.g. not more often than every 20–30 minutes). Acute observation of colour change in the skin, level of consciousness and pulse rate provide all the necessary information in most patients. In some patients continuous recording of arterial pressure throughout anaesthesia and into the recovery period is necessary. This is common after major cardiothoracic surgery or following treatment for major multiple injuries and is achieved by means of an indwelling arterial cannula connected to a pressure transducer and oscilloscope or pen-recording system.

Cardiac irregularities, occurring in the postoperative period, should always be reported to the anaesthetist. Atrial fibrillation may occur following major surgery in elderly patients and its onset is often accompanied by a fall in arterial pressure. Bursts of extrasystoles (dropped-beats) may herald the onset of ventricular fibrillation and cardiac arrest. The precise diagnosis of cardiac irregularities, whatever their cause, usually depends on the e.c.g. and therefore the earlier their occurrence is reported the better.

Venous pressure

The measurement of central venous pressure is frequently made by the anaesthetist in theatre, particularly in cases of severe injuries or during surgery involving a large loss of blood. The central venous pressure is a sensitive index of changes in circulating blood volume and begins to fall before changes in pulse rate or systemic arterial pressure can be detected. Measurements may continue to be made during the recovery period as a guide to further blood or plasma requirements and the nurse should be familiar with the technique of setting up the required apparatus and making the measurements at the appropriate intervals of time.

Figure 9.3 shows the general arrangement of the apparatus. A catheter is passed by the doctor, usually percutaneously, via the internal jugular vein or a convenient arm vein into the superior vena cava. On occasion it may be necessary to perform a formal 'cut-down' on an arm vein or on the saphenous vein at the groin. In the latter case the catheter will be advanced until it lies in the inferior vena cava within the thorax. The catheter is connected to a three-way tap, one arm of which is attached to an intravenous saline infusion and the other to a measuring column calibrated in centimetres of water. The zero on the measuring column must be level with the right atrium whenever a reading is made, i.e. the mid-axillary line when the patient is lying down or the angle of the sternum when sitting up.

A slow infusion is continuously maintained via the catheter except when a measurement is required. At that time the tap is turned to connect the catheter to the measuring column. If the catheter is patent the column of saline should fluctuate with res-

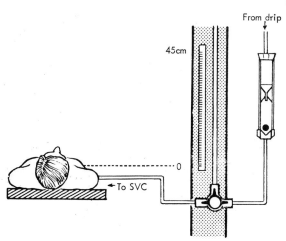

Figure 9.3 A central venous pressure manometer system. The zero point on the scale is levelled with the right atrium.

piration and after allowing a moment or two for the level to settle a reading is made. Normally the central venous pressure should be approximately 6 to 12 centimetres of water. The reading may be higher in right heart failure or overtransfusion or lower when there has been acute haemorrhage or the patient is 'shocked' from another cause. In certain circumstances, measurement of central venous pressure can be misleading because of previous respiratory or cardiac disease and does not truly reflect the pressure in the left atrium and the performance of the heart as a pump. A flow-directed catheter (Swan-Ganz) can be introduced to the right side of the heart via the superior vena cava and when it is wedged in a branch of the pulmonary artery gives a more accurate approximation to the pressure on the left side of the heart. This technique is reserved for patients with major circulatory difficulties in the postoperative period.

Cardiac arrest

The most sudden and dramatic of all emergencies with which the recovery room nurse may have to deal is the occurrence of 'cardiac arrest'. This may follow untreated respiratory inadequacy or a persistent period of hypotension due to any cause, but can frequently occur without warning. Any patients who are especially at risk e.g. those with some degree of heart-block preoperatively, will be indicated to the nurse by anaesthetist. In healthy normal adults, the sensitive nervous tissue of the brain will only survive the results of circulatory standstill and acute hypoxia for a period of about 3 minutes. The immediate recognition of this condition is therefore of the utmost importance if resuscitation is to be successful.

Signs of 'apparent cardiac arrest'

The term 'apparent cardiac arrest' is used deliberately since, if the cardiac action and circulation are so poor that the following signs are present, then immediate treatment is required even if the heart has not quite stopped.
The signs are three in number:
  Pallor or cyanosis of the skin i.e. a sudden deterioration of the skin colour.
  Absence of palpable carotid pulses in the neck. N.B. Not the radial pulses as these are often difficult to feel.

Rapidly dilating pupils. This is a most reliable sign of cerebral hypoxia. Two further secondary signs may be present in appropriate cases. If the patient has been awake, consciousness will be lost quickly and, secondly, respiratory arrest will quickly ensue if cardiac standstill is untreated.

Treatment of cardiac arrest

If these signs are present, immediate action by the recovery room personnel is required. Occasionally this takes the form of direct cardiac massage but more usually external cardiac massage or compression is employed. This is usually sufficient to restore cardiac action and circulation completely. The technique of external cardiac massage is described in Chapter 11.

Gastro-intestinal complications

It is necessary to distinguish between vomiting which is an active process and regurgitation which is a passive and more insidious complication. Regurgitation is seldom accompanied by any outward signs or sounds and occurs when the patient is at a deeper level of unconsciousness, at which time the cough reflexes are less active than normal. Unless adequate precautions have been taken inhalation of the gastric contents will certainly occur. The vomiting patient on the other hand can usually cough vigorously and unless the quantity of vomitus is excessive can expel it safely without danger of inhalation.

These complications are most likely to occur if the stomach has not been emptied adequately before operation, if there was vomiting preoperatively, or if the nature of the illness results in delayed gastric emptying.

Certain anaesthetic agents predispose to nausea and vomiting in the postoperative period, e.g. cyclopropane and ether, but with modern anaesthetic techniques vomiting from this latter cause is uncommon.

Inhalation of gastric contents can result in sudden death from drowning or in acute hypoxia from laryngeal or bronchial spasm. A late result may be the development of pulmonary collapse, pneumonia or lung abscess. One special group of patients, in whom inhalation of foreign material is particularly likely, deserves special mention. When the pharynx and vocal cords have been anaesthetised by topical application of an analgesic agent, e.g. lignocaine 4%, to facilitate endoscopy, the loss of sensation often exceeds the actual operating time by up to 2 hours. Thus no fluids or solids must be given to these patients until the analgesic has ceased to act, lest they are inhaled when the patient attempts to swallow. A simple label on the patient's forehead, drawing attention to the fact that a topical analgesic has been used, is useful in these patients.

Treatment

As always, the best treatment of the condition is prevention. Wherever possible, the stomach should be emptied preoperatively. Even if the gastric tube is left in place after operation, postoperative regurgitation may still take place alongside the tube, particularly if free drainage is not allowed, e.g. if a clamp or spigot is left on the upper end of the tube.

The dangers of vomiting and regurgitation may be lessened to a large extent by the correct posturing of the patient in bed, i.e. the tonsillar position (Fig. 9.4).

If vomiting or regurgitation does occur:

a. Keep the head low. This ensures that all the material will flow out of the mouth and not enter the respiratory tract.

b. Clear the mouth and pharnyx with swabs or suction.

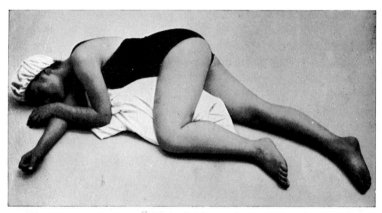

Figure 9.4 The tonsillar position: the patient lies midway between the lateral and the prone positions, prevented from rolling face downwards by the pillow and the position of the arms and legs.

c. Having cleared the airway, ensure that respiration is adequate. If cyanosis persists, administer oxygen.

d. If there is evidence that stomach contents have actually been inhaled more active measures are indicated. Acute pulmonary oedema may follow inhalation of even a small quantity of acid material and requires urgent treatment with oxygen, assisted ventilation, steroid therapy and antibiotics.

Renal complications

Normal renal function is essential to both body water and electrolyte balance and to acid base homeostasis. Impending renal failure may be missed in the immediate postoperative period if there is not a proper understanding of its mechanisms and a recognition of the type of patient who is especially at risk.

Renal failure may be classified as:

1. Pre-renal — this can occur where there is gross dehydration.

2. Post-renal — for example where bilateral calculi obstruct the ureters.

3. Intrinsic — where the renal tissue itself suffers damage which may or may not be reversible.

We are concerned here with pre-renal and instrinsic types. In the pre-renal type of failure which is commonly met with in the surgical patient, treatment consists of the restoration of an adequate circulatory blood volume, replacement of fluid losses and the correction of any electrolyte deficiencies. This will usually result in a return of normal urine flow from the previous oliguric state. Uncorrected or undetected, the pre-renal type of failure can progress to the intrinsic variety which is also known widely as acute tubular necrosis. Failure to achieve a normal urine flow following restoration of the circulatory blood volume usually indicates that intrinsic failure is already established. Even at this stage, the situation may be reversible if a diuretic such as 20% mannitol is given intravenously. Failure to respond to this therapy is an indication for further treatment by the physician which may be conservative or may consist of repeated peritoneal dialysis or haemodialysis to tide the patient over until normal renal function returns.

The predisposing factors are as follows:

1. Reduced renal blood flow due to a reduction in circulating blood, plasma or water and electrolytes.

2. Metabolic acidosis which usually accompanies 'shock'.

3. Excessive circulatory haemoglobin or myoglobin as commonly found in grave multiple injuries.
4. Sepsis.
5. Surgery on the aorta above the level of the renal vessels.

Close observation of the patients in the immediate postoperative period is essential and should consist of hourly urine volume measurement along with blood pressure and central venous pressure measurements. Urine flow is best measured by use of one or other of the 'urinometers' now available (Fig. 9.5). Frequent blood gas analysis is necessary to detect any developing metabolic acidosis as is measurement of the urine and plasma osmolality which gives an indication of the ability of the kidney to concentrate urine.

The initial treatment in a case of early renal failure is outlined below but the early recognition of the condition is of the first importance.

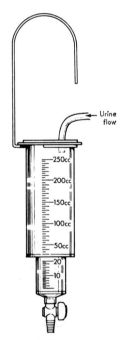

Urine
flow

250cc
200cc
150cc
100cc
50cc
20
10

Figure 9.5 The urinometer illustrated is hooked to a convenient point on the patient's bed. The tap enables the urinometer to be emptied at intervals for biochemical analysis.

Treatment

    a. Maintenance of an adequate circulating blood volume.
    b. Correction of fluid and electrolyte deficiencies.
    c. Intravenous 20% mannitol (two or three doses maximum).

Should this treatment be unavailing, the patient, now in established renal failure, will be managed by the renal physicians and peritoneal dialysis or haemodialysis may ultimately be required.

CARE OF SPECIAL CASES IN THE RECOVERY ROOM

There are additional points to observe in the management of patients who have undergone certain special types of surgery or anaesthesia. These are best considered under separate headings.

1. Epidural and subarachnoid analgesia

These analgesic techniques interfere with three important functions of the recovering patient's normal defence mechanism and this state of affairs often persists well into the recovery period.

Analgesia

The regions of the body, and particularly the skin, served by the nerves which have been blocked as they leave the subarachnoid or epidural space, may still be partially or completely 'anaesthetised' postoperatively. As far as the skin is concerned the patient will not respond normally to pain, heat or cold and damage from pressure or burns is possible.

Reflexes

The normal postural reflexes will be depressed. These reflexes normally prevent over-stretching of muscles or over-extension of joints. Damage can result if the limbs are allowed to remain in abnormal positions for long periods.

    The use of 'ripple mattresses' is of great assistance in the prevention of bed sores in any patient where the one posture is, of necessity, maintained for a long time. An alternative to the ripple mattress is the medical sheepskin. The patient lies on this instead of a mattress and is supported by the cushion of air trapped among the fibres of the material.

Sympathetic blockade

Patients with sympathetic blockade have temporarily lost the normal control of the peripheral blood vessels which helps to maintain the blood pressure at the normal levels. Thus, blood pools in the dependent parts of the body with a resultant severe fall in blood pressure. Therefore, while under the influence of a 'spinal' or epidural analgesic these patients must be nursed in the recumbent position and occasionally in the head-down position until the normal tone returns to their cardiovascular system.

There are certain other points to observe in the management of such cases:

1. Headaches. These not infrequently follow subarachnoid analgesia and their causation is obscure. However, it is well known that headaches are much commoner in patients who have not been nursed in the supine (flat) position for at least 12 hours after the operation.

2. Acute retention of urine. This can occur particularly in older men with some degree of prostatic enlargement. However, the distended bladder does not result in undue discomfort while the analgesic effect persists. The abdomen therefore should be examined regularly for any sign of bladder distension, and catheterisation may be required.

3. Sterility. Particular care must be taken of patients in whom a continuous epidural analgesia is being maintained postoperatively for one reason or another. The nurse may be instructed to make the intermittent injections at certain intervals and *absolute* sterility is mandatory. The technique, using a paediatric intravenous set with burette, to some extent avoids this danger (Fig. 9.6).

2. Induced hypotensive anaesthesia

Some surgical procedures are facilitated if bleeding in the field of operation is reduced to a minimum by lowering the blood pressure deliberately during anaesthesia, e.g. brain surgery, micro-surgery of the middle ear and plastic surgery. This hypotension is usually produced in one of two ways:

a. By epidural or subarachnoid analgesia.

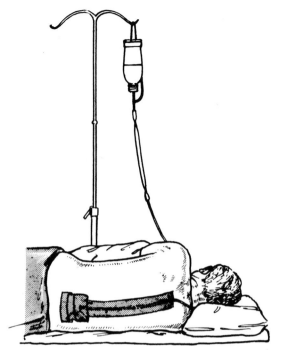

Figure 9.6 An infusion bottle containing the local analgesic solution is shown connected to the epidural catheter by a paediatric drip set. In this way small supplementary doses of solution can be administered to maintain analgesia both during and after operation. The epidural catheter is secured along the patient's back with adhesive strapping over a sterile dressing.

b. By the intravenous injection of ganglion blocking drugs like trimetaphan (Arfonad) or sodium nitroprusside (Nipride).

The loss of vasomotor tone (i.e. dilatation of the blood vessels) produced by these methods may last well into the recovery room phase, and, although the patient may have become fully conscious, he is still very likely to suffer a severe fall in blood pressure if allowed to sit up. Frequent pulse and blood pressure recording is therefore of the greatest importance in all these patients, until the drug effect wears off.

3. Induced hypothermia

This technique is usually confined to cardiovascular and neurosurgical procedures, or following severe head injuries. The management of patients suffering from malignant hyperpyrexia also involves the active cooling of the patient as an important part of the emergency treatment. The patient's body temperature is lowered to between 29°C and 32°C (normal body temperature 37°C) and active rewarming of such cases is carried out in the recovery room until the body temperature is about 36°C. This rewarming process is carried out with electric blankets, special mattresses which contain circulating warm water, or by a fan blowing warm air over the body surface. Although this process is always closely supervised by the anaesthetist, the recovery room nurse has an important part to play. The recording of temperature at frequent intervals, in addition to pulse, blood pressure and respiratory rate, is usually the responsibility of the nurse. A few words of explanation about temperature recording in these cases may be useful at this point.

'Body' temperature is a meaningless phrase unless the site at which the recording is made is indicated, e.g. rectum, oesophagus, nasopharynx or axilla. Commonly the rectal or oesophageal temperature is monitored during rewarming and specially designed continuously recording thermometers are used for the purpose, since the usual mercury clinical thermometer is not suitable (Fig. 9.7). The thermometer is read at frequent intervals, e.g. 5 minutes, until a return to normal is achieved.

Special attention must be paid to the skin during rewarming to avoid contact burns and pressure sores.

4. Endoscopies

The diagnostic procedures of laryngoscopy, bronchoscopy and oesophagoscopy are frequently carried out under topical analgesia, with or without a general anaesthetic being given as well. Lignocaine in a 4% solution is often employed and its analgesic action can last up to 2 hours. During this period there is a loss of sensation in the mouth, oropharynx and larynx and no cough reflex is present. It is obvious that two dangers have to be avoided in the recovery room:

    a. Any solids given orally may enter the lungs.
    b. Hot liquids may cause burns to the anaesthetised area.

For a period of at least 3 hours from the start of anaesthesia, no fluids or solids are given to these patients despite the fact that they may be fully conscious and co-operative.

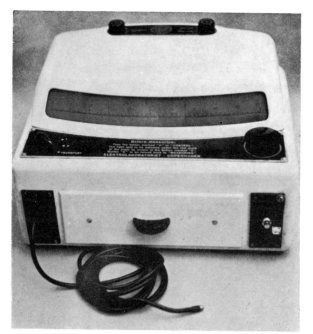

Figure 9.7 A recording thermometer with an oesophageal lead attached.

Due to the absence of the cough reflex, secretions tend to accumulate in the mouth and airway and these patients must be encouraged to cough them up or, if necessary, they must be removed by the nurse with gentle suction. The use of the tonsillar position in bed, even when the patient is fully conscious, has much to recommend it.

5. Restless patients

Restlessness, in the patient recovering from anaesthesia, is a common finding and the diagnosis and treatment of the underlying cause is worthy of special mention. Too often restlessness is interpreted only as a need for a sedative or analgesic. It is essential that the cause be accurately identified and *no* sedation must be given until this has been done. The following are some of the possible causes of postoperative restlessness:

a. *Inadequate respiration.* This can be diagnosed with certainty if signs of hypoxia or carbon dioxide retention are present (see p. 76).

b. Haemorrhage. A fall in blood pressure with tachycardia is strongly suggestive of hidden bleeding.

c. Pain other then wound pain. This may result from a full bladder or pins in the dressings puncturing the skin etc.

6. Post-thoracotomy patients

Certain complications may occur in patients who have undergone the operation of thoracotomy. The two most dangerous in the postoperative period are unrecognised bleeding inside the chest resulting in a *haemothorax,* or air inside the chest escaping from a damaged area of lung resulting in *pneumothorax.* The presence of blood or air in quantity within the pleural cavity causes collapse of the underlying lung with the development of inadequate respiration. Because of these dangers a drain is usually inserted by the surgeon into the pleural cavity at the end of the operation. If this were an ordinary tube drain such as is commonly used following abdominal surgery, air would be sucked into the chest during inspiration and the lung would collapse.

There are three variations of the water-sealed drain in common use. The first of these is illustrated in Figure 9.8 and is the method most commonly employed. Where large quantities of blood or fluid are expected, a second collecting bottle can be interposed between the water-seal bottle and the patient. This enables a more precise measurement of the blood loss to be made when the collecting bottle is suitably calibrated.

The third method of drainage is used in situations where it is desirable to be able to control the .negative pressure within the water-sealed system to keep the lung fully expanded (Figs. 9.9, 9.10). This time the second bottle is on the opposite side of the water-sealed bottle from the patient and has an additional tube open to atmosphere at one end and submerged 5 to 10 cm below the surface of the sterile liquid at the other. Adjustment of this tube at different depths below the surface maintains the negative pressure with the whole system at −5 to −10 cm H_2O. It is possible to attach this bottle to suction apparatus and this is usually done where there is a large air-leak from the lung such as is encountered in bronchopleural fistula. The application of a dangerously large negative pressure to the pleural cavity is avoided since, if the −5 to −10 cm selected pressure is exceeded, air will be drawn into the system from the atmosphere via the open end of the third tube. When suction is

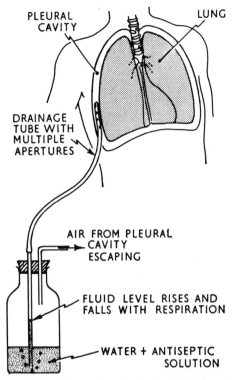

PLEURAL
CAVITY

LUNG

DRAINAGE
TUBE WITH
MULTIPLE
APERTURES

AIR FROM PLEURAL
CAVITY
ESCAPING

FLUID LEVEL RISES AND
FALLS WITH RESPIRATION

WATER + ANTISEPTIC
SOLUTION

Figure 9.8 Water-seal drain: It is important that the chest drain be attached to the glass tube which opens under the surface of the liquid in the bottle.

used in this way, air should always be seen to be bubbling gently from the submerged end of the tube.

Although the intrathoracic catheter is generally inserted so that it lies in the lower part of the pleural cavity when blood and fluid are being drained, an apical drain is best where air is leaking from the lung. The reason for employing the higher position is that air collects in the upper pleural cavity if the patient is semi-recumbent or erect.

A word of warning is necessary when moving these patients. During transportation of the patient or moving him about in bed the bottle must always be kept at a *lower* level than the chest, unless the tubing is clamped, otherwise the fluid in the bottle will flow back up the tube into the chest. If the chest drain is patent the level of the fluid in the descending glass tube will fluctuate smoothly with respiration. If it does not, then the tube is probably blocked with

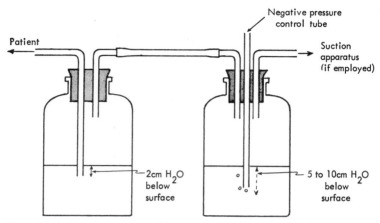

Figure 9.9 A water-seal system enabling the negative pressure to be adjusted as required.

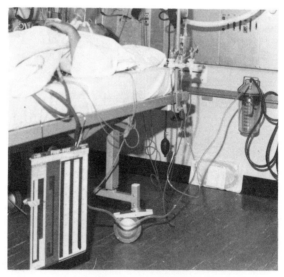

Figure 9.10 Pleur-evac disposable system for underwater-seal drainage of the pleural cavity. There are three integral components: (1) suction control chamber; (2) water seal chamber; (3) calibrated drainage collection chamber. The system is connected to the piped suction system via a reservoir mounted on the wall rail.

debris or clotted blood and must be gently 'milked' until patent again. Alternatively, a one-way valve may be attached to the chest drain (Fig. 9.11).

Although a chest drain is usually introduced to the pleural cavity

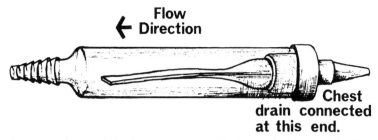

Figure 9.11 The Heimlich valve. This one-way valve is interposed between the chest drain and the drainage bottle. Air and blood may flow in the direction indicated but the rubber valve prevents air entering the pleural cavity.

formally during open thoracotomy there are occasions in emergency situations where a catheter has to be introduced quickly by a 'blind' technique. This is done where there has been a rapid and dangerous accumulation of air or blood in the pleural cavity often after an injury to the chest. The catheter may be placed at the base or the apex of the cavity and this is done usually under local analgesia, by means of a trochar which is inserted within the catheter. Through a small skin incision the trochar and catheter are advanced between the ribs until the pleural cavity is penetrated. The trochar is then removed and the catheter connected to the water-seal drainage bottle in the usual way. In order to facilitate positioning of the catheter it has a radio-opaque strip along its length which enables it to be seen clearly on X-ray (Fig. 9.12).

Patients who have had a thoracic operation may have a considerable amount of wound pain and pleural irritation from the chest drain. This discourages them from moving, breathing deeply or coughing. Of course, this results in retention of secretions in the bronchi and leads to hypoxia and carbon dioxide retention. Adequate doses of analgesics must be given to permit a good respiratory effort to be maintained and coughing must be encouraged to clear the airway of secretions. Nowhere is the value of the postoperative recovery room more apparent than in the supervision of these patients.

7. Post-craniotomy patients

The postoperative care of patients who have undergone neurosurgical procedures is worthy of special mention. These patients may be conscious or unconscious. In the case of the conscious patient

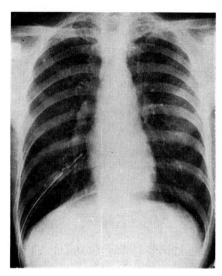

Figure 9.12 An Argyle thoracic catheter in position showing the radio-opaque marker.

the problem usually resolves itself into the careful observation of the conscious level, the cardiopulmonary state and the ensuring of adequate nutrition. Where the patient is unconscious, meticulous attention must be paid to alterations in the level of consciousness and for this purpose a special chart is of assistance (p. 121). Signs of increased intracranial pressure are an indication for urgent intervention to avoid irreparable cerebral damage from 'coning'. The measurement of central venous pressure is invaluable as an uncontrolled rise will result in increased intracranial pressure.

The management of the airway in those patients is as always of paramount importance since hypoxaemia or carbon dioxide retention can increase cerebral oedema and prejudice the patient's recovery. The use of naso-tracheal tubes is of great assistance here and reduces the need for tracheostomy. Active cooling measures may be required where hyperthermia is a complication.

OXYGEN THERAPY

The gas most commonly utilised in inhalation therapy is oxygen, although mixtures of oxygen with carbon dioxide (in carbon monoxide poisoning) or helium (in respiratory obstruction) are occasionally used. Increasing the concentration of oxygen, even to

100% in the inspired gas or air is of limited value if respiratory obstruction or inadequate respiration is present. Where hypoxia is present and oxygen therapy instituted the person who initiates this treatment must ensure that the airway is clear and ventilation adequate—or should seek help. Delivering 100% oxygen to the face of an apnoeic patient without ensuring a clear airway and manually or mechanically assisting ventilation is futile.

Rationale of oxygen therapy

Ambient air contains approximately 21% oxygen at a partial pressure of about 150 mm Hg (20 kPa) (1/5 of 760 mm Hg or 101.5 kPa). When a patient breathes 100% oxygen the nitrogen in the lungs is 'washed' out and the partial pressure of oxygen in the lungs is increased to nearly 760 mm Hg (101.5 kPa). Thus the pressure gradient for oxygen diffusion across the alveolar capillary membrane is greatly increased, more oxygen is dissolved in the plasma and the plasma content is increased ten fold, i.e. from 0.3 ml O_2/100 ml plasma to 3 ml/100 ml plasma. It is apparent that any further increase in the plasma content of oxygen can only be achieved by raising the ambient pressure above normal. This is a technique which requires a pressure chamber and those in cur-rent use raise the ambient pressure from 1 atmosphere (760 mm Hg or 101.5 kPa) to 2 and for some purposes 3 atmospheres. At 3 atmospheres the plasma content of oxygen is increased to 5.6 ml O_2/100 ml plasma which is almost sufficient to maintain life without the oxygen linked to haemoglobin, since around 5 ml O_2/100 ml blood is the basic metabolic requirement.

Toxic effects of oxygen therapy

1. In patients with respiratory disease depending on 'anoxic drive' to the respiratory centre to maintain respiration, uncontrolled oxygen administration can lead to respiratory depression and even apnoea.

2. Prolonged oxygen therapy results in vasoconstriction and in neonates leads to retrolental fibroplasia if concentrations greater than 40% are administered.

3. Pulmonary damage with oedema may follow prolonged ad-ministration of 100% oxygen.

4. Prolonged exposure to 100% oxygen at raised ambient press-ures (2-3 atmospheres) can cause disturbance to the central nervous

system with convulsions. In addition severe pain in the air sinuses and middle ear may occur.

Methods of administration

There are four main methods of oxygen administration.

1. Nasal catheter. This method is of use where only a modest increase in the inspired oxygen concentration is desired. Low flows of about 3 litres/minute are well tolerated by the patient and this gives an inspired oxygen concentration of about 25%.

2. Masks. Many differing types of mask are now available, plastic disposable ones being most popular. Higher flow rates are tolerated by the patient but the flow rate must never be less than the patient's minute volume or rebreathing and carbon dioxide retention will occur. The average adult requires a flow of at least 8 litres oxygen/minute which will give an inspired oxygen concentration of 50–60%.

3. Venturi masks. This type of mask, making use of the Venturi principle, enables the physician to control more accurately the oxygen concentration administered to the patient. Thus oxygen can be administered to patients with hypoxic drive with less risk of respiratory depression.

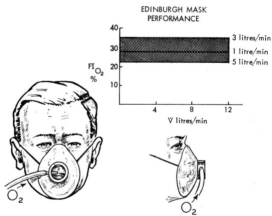

Figure 9.13 The Edinburgh Mask. The inset graph shows the percentage of oxygen in the inspired gas mixture (FI_{O_2}%) achieved by delivering different flow rates of oxygen to the open-ended mask. It can be seen that the percentage of oxygen breathed by the patient varies little with changes in the minute volume (V litres/minute). (*After* Flenley, D. C., Hutchison, D. C. S. & Donald, K. W. (1963) *British Medical Journal* 2, 1081).

4. Oxygen tents. This method is now not so popular as formerly. The tent makes nursing difficult and many patients become claustrophobic. Continual opening and closing of the tent to permit nursing procedures results in practice in low oxygen concentrations.

Oxygen as a vehicle for drug administration

Bronchodilator drugs such as isoprenaline can be administered in a fine droplet suspension in oxygen using a nebuliser attachment to the administration apparatus. This technique is useful in patients with bronchospasm particularly when combined with the inhalation of mucolytic agents such as chymotrypsin or Alevaire to liquefy the tenacious sputum. Antibiotics may also be administered in this way although it is more logical and efficient to give them by injection.

Control of oxygen therapy

It would quite reasonably be thought rash if a clinician were to administer a potent drug from an uncalibrated syringe. Oxygen is a widely used drug and its safe and effective administration requires similar control. Such control implies measurements of two kinds. Firstly, measurement of the dose administered to the patient and secondly, measurement of the effect of the drug on the patient's condition. The following are the various ways in which oxygen administration can be controlled.

1. Methods of measuring amount of oxygen delivered

Flowmeter. This device measures in litres/minute the flow of oxygen delivered to the patient.

Oxygen analyser. Different types of analyser are available for sampling the inspired concentration (F_1O_2) breathed by the patient from mask or ventilator. This measurement should be made at the same time as the patient's arterial oxygen saturation and tension are measured in order to relate one to the other.

2. Methods of assessing therapy in patients

Colour of skin and mucosae. This is unreliable since hypoxaemia can exist in the absence of cyanosis. In addition, lighting conditions and the state of the patient's peripheral circulation can lead to erroneous assessment.

Oximetry. Apparatus is available which measures the arterial haemoglobin oxygen saturation indirectly by detecting the changes in light reflection through the patient's capillary bed, e.g. in the ear-lobe. This method is imprecise where the peripheral circulation is poor.

Arterial oxygen measurement. This is the most accurate technique. An arterial blood sample is used and the percentage saturation of the haemoglobin with oxygen (Sa_{o2}) and the arterial oxygen tension (Pa_{o2}) estimated. To facilitate repeated measurements in acute illness, indwelling arterial cannulae may be employed.

SEDATIVES, ANALGESICS AND HYPNOTICS

An important part of the after-care of patients is the provision of adequate sedation or analgesia where anxiety or pain is present. By definition, to sedate means to soothe or settle, but it is customary to use the term sedative to describe drugs which relieve anxiety while the terms analgesic and hypnotic are correctly applied to pain-relieving and sleep-producing agents, respectively.

There is often an overlap in the actions of a drug, some analgesics, notably the opiates, relieving anxiety, and many sedatives, for example the barbiturates, in larger doses inducing sleep. It is therefore essential in selecting the appropriate drug to decide whether the aim is to remedy pain, anxiety or restlessness. It must be remembered also that if a drug is prescribed within a few hours of the beginning or end of an operation it may interact with other drugs used during anaesthesia, producing deeper or longer sleep than expected and/or more severe depression of blood pressure or respiration than is desirable. For the safety of the patient, the house officer and anaesthetist usually co-operate in deciding which drugs are to be given immediately before and after operation.

Pain relief

If pain is present an analgesic should be administered. For milder or more chronic pain one may use tablets of codeine or paracetamol, 1 to 2, orally, 4-hourly. Pain of greater severity may respond to dihydrocodeine bitartrate (DF 118), 30 to 60 mg, or pentazocine, 50 to 70 mg, by mouth.

For severe pain, particularly in the postoperative period, the opiates or pethidine are still the drugs of choice. Morphine sulphate, 10 to 15 mg, papaveretum, 10 to 20 mg, or pethidine, 50 to 100 mg, can be given parenterally for the average adult patient (70 kg body weight). Pentazocine, 20 to 30 mg, may also be used. Pentazocine is claimed to be a non-addictive analgesic and is related to the opiate antagonist nalorphine. Its duration of action is shorter than that of morphine but the incidence of emetic sequelae is also considerably lower. In a further attempt to reduce the incidence of nausea and vomiting, narcotic analgesics may be given along with an anti-emeric drug such as promethazine, one of the phenothiazine group. This combination also enhances the sedative effect of the analgesic.

There are obvious advantages in the postoperative period of ensuring prolonged and effective pain relief with the minimum number of injections. A new potent analgesic buprenorphine (Temgesic), which has recently been introduced to clinical practice, can provide excellent analgesia for periods in excess of 8 hours. A dose of 0.3 mg is approximately equivalent to 10 mg morphine and the drug may be administered intravenously, intramuscularly or sublingually. The same effect of course may be achieved by the continuous intravenous infusion of a drug such as morphine by means of a syringe pump, the dosage rate being adjusted according to the patient's needs. It should be emphasised that this technique is really only suitable where skilled supervision can be guaranteed at all times. In selecting the correct dose of any analgesic consideration should be given to the patient's physical state, his weight and any other drugs given recently. Many anaesthetists give the first postoperative dose of analgesic in dilute solution intravenously, e.g. morphine 10 mg, or pethidine 100 mg in 10 ml water, taking several minutes to complete the injection and stopping the injection when pain is relieved. This technique is best employed initially under supervision. The opiates provide better psychic sedation than pethidine and in equi-analgesic doses (morphine 10 mg = pethidine 60 to 65 mg) there is little difference in side-effects, i.e. respiratory depression and nausea and vomiting. Papaveretum is claimed to produce less respiratory depression and nausea than morphine because of the papaverine content but in equi-analgesic dosage with morphine the degree of respiratory and cardiovascular depression is similar. The respiratory depression produced by all three drugs may be antagonised by the intravenous injection of nalorphine 5 to 10 mg, levallorphan, 1 to 2 mg, or naloxone, 0.5 mg. Care must be taken not to overshoot the dose of the first two of these drugs necessary to reverse the respiratory depression present since the effect is then to increase the depression. The use of a premixed combination of pethidine and levallorphan (100 mg : 1.25 mg) has little to recommend it except that it serves to remind all concerned that they are dealing with a patient who is liable to develop respiratory insufficiency.

Relief of anxiety may help to relieve pain and the use of the benzodiazepines is of value. Bear in mind also the value of reassurance and attention to bodily comfort—keeping the patient warm for example. Also of immense value is some form of distraction such as conversation with other patients. Finally, for painful dressings premixed nitrous oxide and oxygen as used in labour (p. 68) may be employed. It may be used also to supplement narcotic therapy preceding and during physiotherapy.

Anxiety

This is a common occurrence in a hospital ward and one which is all too often ignored. Many studies have shown that a patient who approaches surgery in an anxious state requires much more postoperative analgesia. Explanation, reassurance and the administration of diazepam or other anxiolytic drugs are all very worth while.

Insomnia

There are a vast number of hypnotics from which to choose. Many patients may already have been in the habit to taking such drugs at home and it is often wise to continue the same agent if it has been having a good effect. For the remainder, nitrazepam (5 to 10 mg) is considered by many to be the safest hypnotic for long-term use. Of the barbiturates, pentobarbitone, quinalbarbitone, butobarbitone and amylobarbitone (100 to 200 mg of any orally) all have their advocates. These are best avoided in the elderly in case they cause confusion; glutethimide (Doriden), 250 to 500 mg, or methaqualone, 150 to 300 mg, orally are useful alternatives.

Not all hypnotics are equally effective in different individuals and one must be prepared to change if necessary. Many patients lie awake due to worry which could be largely relieved by daytime anxiolytic therapy.

Restlessness

Restlessness may be associated with pain in the patient recovering from anaesthesia but not yet fully conscious. This restlessness usually responds to an analgesic. In the conscious patient it may be associated with anxiety, in which case it responds to a barbiturate or tranquilliser. *Restlessness may be associated with inadequate respiration or concealed haemorrhage* and these must be excluded as the injudicious use of sedatives may be lethal in such cases. In other cases restlessness is associated with head injury or is found in older patients. Promazine or chlorpromazine, 25 to 50 mg orally or intramuscularly, is of value in some of these cases but a specialist opinion is usually desirable before treating a restless patient where the cause is not obvious.

Paraldehyde, 10 to 15 ml orally or rectally or up to 0.2 mg/kg intramuscularly, should be reserved for otherwise uncontrollable patients.

The following important points are well worth emphasising:

Always use a drug appropriate to the symptoms being treated—analgesics for pain, hypnotics for insomnia, etc.

Learn to use a small number of effective drugs.

When dealing with restless patients always try to identify the cause before treatment.

Keep a clear record of all drugs given, their dosage, route, time of administration and effect. This record is invaluable as a guide to others before further drugs are prescribed.

10

The respiratory
intensive care unit

The postoperative recovery phase usually lasts from 1 to 24 hours. However, certain patients may require much longer special care and they are best accommodated in an intensive care unit, where other patients, not necessarily postoperative, are intensively nursed for longer periods of time, e.g. 2 days to 6 weeks.

This pattern of progressive care of patients throughout their stay in hospital can be applied more widely than to surgical patients alone. Figure 10.1 demonstrates schematically the various pathways the patient may follow after reception at an emergency admission unit until his ultimate discharge from hospital. In any individual case the sole consideration which determines the patient's place of treatment is the degree of observation and the amount of therapy required. The most ill patients are, therefore, gathered together in areas where staff and equipment are concentrated to enable intensive observation and therapy to be undertaken. Intensive care areas are made up of individual units restricted to the treatment of a particular group of patients, such as those suffering from respiratory or renal failure and myocardial infarction.

The anaesthetist is mainly concerned with that part of the intensive care area where patients with respiratory problems are treated, and it is this type of patient whom we shall consider here. The following are some of the conditions which can lead to a

RESUSCITATION & PROGRESSIVE CARE

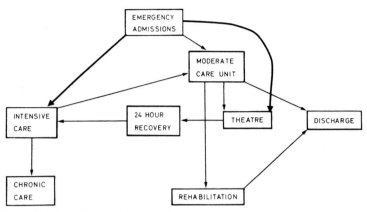

Figure 10.1 Resuscitation and progressive care.

patient's admission to the Respiratory Intensive Care Unit:
1. Postoperative respiratory insufficiency.
2. Severe head injuries and facio-maxillary injuries.
3. Trauma to the chest wall: crushed-chest injuries.
4. Obstructive lung disease with respiratory failure (emphysema with an additional acute respiratory infection).
5. Carbon monoxide poisoning and drug overdose.
6. Certain infectious diseases: poliomyelitis, polyneuritis, tetanus.
7. Miscellaneous medical conditions: cerebrovascular accidents, myasthenia gravis, acute porphyria.

A proportion of patients admitted to the intensive care unit will require mainly simple supportive measures and controlled oxygen therapy while they are the subject of continuous observation. The majority, however, will require more vigorous treatment and in particular measures aimed at augmenting their own inadequate respiratory effort and specific therapy.

SPECIAL PROCEDURES IN THE RESPIRATORY UNIT

The methods and manoeuvres used in the recovery room are, of course, also practised in the respiratory unit, but a knowledge of some additional procedures is essential.

1. Parenteral feeding

Particular attention should be paid to the nutritional requirements of all patients from the time of admission to the intensive care unit. So far as post-traumatic and postoperative patients are concerned, it is very common for a metabolic or nutritional problem to be revealed as a major factor in their illness although all these patients have been admitted primarily as respiratory problems.

The two commoner potential causes of starvation in these patients are *excessive catabolism*, or breakdown of tissue, following injury or major surgery and *malabsorption* from the gastro-intestinal tract where there is some degree of paralytic ileus. Both factors may be operative and be further aggravated by the presence of sepsis. A fully balanced diet of adequate calorific content and containing sufficient protein should be given by mouth wherever possible to suit the individual requirements. (See Appendix 1.) If the patient cannot swallow then this diet can be liquefied and given with a naso-gastric tube. If this is not attainable within a few hours of admission then full intravenous feeding is instituted. Solutions of essential amino-acids are available, the building materials from

A. Intravenous diet for a 24-hour period for a 70 kg adult.

Solution	Volume (ml)	Calories	Nitrogen content (grams/litre)
Amino-acids (e.g. Trophysan (conc.) 10%)	1000	724	12.8
Fat emulsion (e.g. Lipiphysan 10%)	500	620	0
Carbohydrate (e.g. Sorbitol 30%)	1500	1800	0
Total	3000	3144	12.8

Note: The fat and amino-acid solutions are usually given simultaneously with the sugar solution using a 'Y' drip. One bottle of carbohydrate (500 ml) can be replaced by a bottle of normal saline or other electrolyte solution if required. Other electrolyte supplements, e.g. potassium, are given as required, as also are vitamin supplements.

B. Intravenous diet for a 24-hour period for a 20 kg child.

Solution	Volume (ml)	Calories	Nitrogen content (grams/litre)
Amino-acids (e.g. Trophysan 5%)	500	182	6.68
Fat emulsion (e.g. Lipiphysan 10%)	250	310	0
Carbohydrate (e.g. Sorbitol 30%)	250	300	0
Total	1000	792	7

Note: Additional fluid requirements can be met by adding dextrose/water or half-strength normal saline in appropriate volume. Vitamin and electrolyte supplements must also be added.

which tissue proteins are constructed in the body, and also solutions of intravenous fats and concentrated sugars, to provide the calorific energy required for metabolism in general and tissue repair in particular. These solutions are hypertonic and are therefore best given via a large vein, usually the superior or inferior vena cava. If peripheral veins are used then the site of infusion must frequently be changed to avoid thrombophlebitis developing.

Particular care is required when administering intravenous fat emulsions since some patients may produce an allergic type reaction requiring the discontinuing of the infusion and the administration of an antihistamine such as chlorpheniramine maleake (Piriton). Fat emulsions are also contraindicated in pregnancy, liver disease and where there is a blood disease with an increased bleeding tendency. Nevertheless, the ability to provide full nutritional requirements parenterally is a most valuable therapeutic measure in the intensive care of these severely ill patients. Two diets are listed on page 104, one suitable for an adult and one for a child requiring intravenous feeding.

2. Tracheostomy

If assistance to ventilation is required it is usually necessary to do this with an endotracheal tube in place. This enables secretions in the bronchi to be aspirated by suction and usually guarantees an unobstructed airway. The endotracheal tube is a temporary expedient and is not commonly left in place beyond a few days. If treatment is required for longer periods then it is usual to perform a tracheostomy.

Indications. Although the operation is apparently performed for many varying surgical and medical conditions these fall readily into two main groups:

a. Conditions in which there is obstruction to the patient's airway, particularly in its upper part, e.g. acute odema of the glottis and carcinoma of larynx. The value of tracheostomy is obvious here—the obstruction is bypassed and free and tranquil respiration ensues.

b. The second group of conditions, where tracheostomy is indicated, is the one in which impairment of the patient's respiratory function, other than simple airway obstruction, is a threat to life. The causes of respiratory insufficiency (Ch. 9) have already been dealt with and may vary from acute trauma to poliomyelitis.

Such patients have usually either no cough or, at the best, an ineffective one and secretions rapidly accumulate in the airway and must be removed.

Advantages of tracheostomy

1. Some reduction of the dead-space formed by the upper air passages results and may marginally improve alveolar ventilation.
2. Easier removal of secretions from the air passages.
3. A reduction in the work of ventilation and in oxygen requirements results from 1 and 2.
4. Better control of oxygen administration is possible via a tracheostomy box and humidifier (Figs. 10.4 and 10.5).
5. In patients with depressed cough and swallowing reflexes, the lungs can be sealed off.
6. Should mechanical assistance to ventilation be required, in addition, this is facilitated by a tracheostomy.

Management of tracheostomy (see also Appendix)

In order that the patient may benefit fully from this procedure certain problems of management must be understood and overcome.

a. *Care of tubes.* It is customary to insert a tube through the tracheostomy opening into the trachea. Anaesthetists use one of the cuffed variety, as this type of tube provides an effective seal for the lungs from secretions and makes possible assisted or controlled ventilation, should this be required. Overinflation of the cuff for long periods can lead to excessive pressure on the tracheal mucosa and to necrosis and sloughing. This complication can be avoided by correct inflation of the cuff to make a seal without excessive pressure and, perhaps, by deflation of the cuff at intervals. Deflation of the cuff must always be preceded by thorough oropharyngeal suction so that any secretions will not run down alongside the tube into the lungs. A double-cuffed tube (the Rüsch tube) may further reduce these hazards in that the two cuffs can be alternately deflated and inflated to reduce the chances of mucosal ulceration but at no time are the lungs entirely without protection. Tubes must be changed frequently since the inside becomes encrusted with dried secretions, particularly when the sputum is copious and viscid. The lumen of the tube gradually becomes blocked and death from acute asphyxia may result. These tubes are usually changed at least every 48 hours.

After use, the tube must be cleaned in the same way as an endotracheal tube and autoclaved, before being used again. It is obvious that if disposable tracheostomy tubes are employed, the problems of cleaning and sterilisation are circumvented (Fig. 10.2).

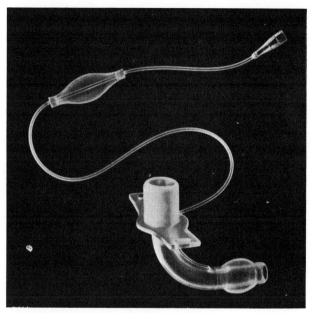

Figure 10.2 The Portex disposable tracheostomy tube.

b. Humidification. Since the paranasal sinuses and nasopharynx, whose function is to warm and humidify the inspired air, have been bypassed by the tracheostomy, it is necessary to provide an alternative source of moisture and heat, to avoid hardening of the secretions and drying and fissuring of the mucosa of the respiratory tract. This can be done in various ways:

(i) It may be sufficient to inject small quantities (e.g. 0.5 ml) of sterile saline down the tracheostomy tube at intervals.

(ii) If the patient is breathing room air, then, in our humid British climate, it is often sufficient to conserve the moisture in the patient's own expirations with a simple condenser humidifier (Fig. 10.3). The moisture in each expiration condenses on the wire-mesh and revaporises on inspiration. These condenser humidifiers are

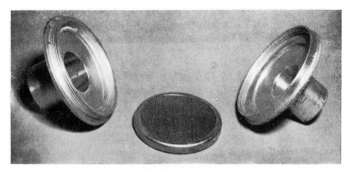

Figure 10.3 The Condenser humidifier: the two parts of the humidifier have been unscrewed to reveal the removable wire-gauze insert.

efficient only when the mesh remains reasonably dry and so they must be changed repeatedly, usually 3 hourly, and dried. The wire-mesh also serves to trap large dust particles and prevent their inhalation.

(iii) In a dry climate, where the atmosphere contains little water vapour, or when the patient breathes oxygen, which is delivered free of moisture and fairly cold from the cylinder or pipe-line, active warming and humidification is usually required. This is done by passing the oxygen or air/oxygen mixture through a 'tank' type humidifier (Fig. 10.4) which warms the gas to about body temperature and saturates it with water-vapour. The warm and moist oxygen then passes along a tube to a tracheostomy box or a plastic 'T'

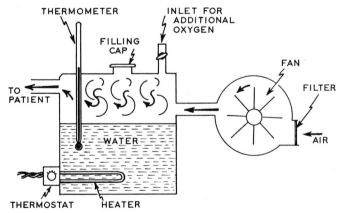

Figure 10.4 The tank humidifier: air or air and oxygen are blown over the surface of the warm water and then to the patient.

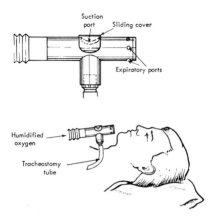

Figure 10.5 A tracheostomy T piece.

piece mounted on the tracheostomy tube (Fig. 10.3). The tracheostomy box or 'T' piece has a series of holes in its surface to permit free expiration and elimination of carbon dioxide which would otherwise accumulate. There is also a port-hole, with a cover which slides to one side, to give access for endotracheal suction.

(iv) There are other devices designed to solve the problem of humidification and these act like perfume 'atomisers' and spray a fine mist of water droplets into the stream of air or oxygen as it is inspired. These devices have the advantage that bronchodilator drugs, e.g. isoprenaline (Neo-epinine), salbutamol (Ventolin) or antibiotics may be suspended in the water and delivered into the depths of the lungs.

Before leaving the problem of humidification it is necessary to mention, if only to condemn, the practice of 'humidifying' oxygen by passing it through a Wolff's bottle. The bubbles which result may serve to amuse the nurse and distract the patient, but the device is valueless as a means of adding sufficient moisture to the inspired gases.

c. Endobronchial suction. The care with which secretions are aspirated from the patient's airway is of the greatest importance. The accent should always be on sterility, thoroughness and gentleness.

It is obvious that the patient is at risk from whatever lethal organism is carelessly introduced due to inadequate sterile technique. If not of the disposable type the endobronchial catheters should be used only once and then cleaned and autoclaved. The catheter used for oropharyngeal suction should not then be used for suction through the tracheostomy. The nurse's hands should be scrubbed before each period of suction and even then should never come in contact with that portion of the catheter which enters the patient's airway.

Endotracheal suction should be carried out as often as is necessary to keep the airways free from secretions. The more copious the secretions, the more often must the manoeuvre be repeated. Whenever possible two people should co-operate during this time, one carrying out the aspiration and the other turning the patient from one side to the other to ensure that the catheter enters both right and left main bronchi.

It is a valuable guide to the adequacy of air-entry in both lungs following suction if the nurse has been taught to listen over both lung fields with a stethoscope. Gross differences in air-entry are readily detected and are an indication for further physiotherapy and endo-bronchial suction.

The size of the catheter selected is important. It should never be thicker than half the diameter of the tracheostomy tube, otherwise it will partially or completely block it and result in acute asphyxia. The catherer should be nipped between finger and thumb when first introduced and released to allow suction only on withdrawal, otherwise there is real danger that excessive suction will collapse portions of the lung. The negative suction pressure should never be greater than is required to remove the secretions easily. More powerful suction is, of course, required when the sputum is thick and tenacious. At all times, the catheter should be handled gently to avoid unnecessary trauma to the sensitive mucosa of the respiratory tract.

Complications of tracheostomy

1. *Infection.* Tracheostomy opens up a route for secondary infection of the lungs and hence the management of such cases must be attended by scrupulous aseptic precautions.

2. *Loss of humidification.* Loss of the normal humidification of the inspired gases by the paranasal sinuses and nasopharynx results in crusting of secretions in the airway.

3. *Mucosal ulceration.* Due to excessive pressure in the tracheostomy tube cuff.

4. *Dilatation of the trachea.* Overinflation of the tube cuff can, on occasion, result in erosion of the cartilaginous rings of the trachea and resultant dilatation.

5. *Granuloma.* Trauma to the tracheal muscosa can lead to the development of granulation tissue and a small polyp may result.

6. *Fistula formation.* This is a serious complication which may occur rarely. Excessive cuff pressure and other trauma leads to the formation of a tracheo-oesophegeal fistula. Food and secretions enter the trachea below the cuff of the tube and contaminate the lungs.

7. *Sinus formation.* Imperfect healing of the post-tracheostomy stoma can result in persistent sinus requiring surgical closure.

8. *Erosion of blood vessels.* Particularly if the stoma becomes infected, a blood vessel may be eroded by the tracheostomy tube and give rise to severe haemorrhage.

9. *Tracheal stricture.* In some 2% of patients with tracheostomy, who have had ventilator treatment, a stricture may develop either at the site of the cuff or at the lower end of the tube. This is a serious late complication often requiring difficult plastic surgery. It is commoner in young children where the cross-section of the airway is quite small. Nasotracheal intubation is preferred to tracheostomy in children to avoid this.

3. Mechanical assistance to ventilation (intermittent positive pressure ventilation: IPPV)

There are two main groups of patients outside of the operating room who require mechanical assistance to ventilation:

Those with demonstrable respiratory failure from whatever cause.

Those patients in whom the development of respiratory failure may confidently be anticipated. Examples of this group are patients with gross cardiopulmonary disease who undergo emergency surgery, extremely obese patients in the postoperative period and patients with gross metabolic disturbance. Ventilators produce a rhythmic inflation and deflation of the patient's lung by intermittently delivering gases at a pressure above atmospheric pressure by way of a face-mask, endotracheal tube or tracheostomy tube (Fig. 10.6). In a sense, they act as another pair of hands, squeezing the bellows for the anaesthetist. The apparatus may vary from the relatively simple manual resuscitators of the Ambu type to

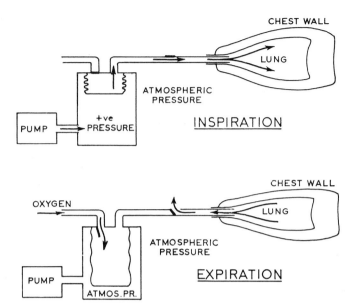

Figure 10.6 Diagram of ventilator action. The bellows or bag containing the fresh gases is enclosed in an airtight chamber and squeezed during inspiration by the action of a pump which raises the pressure inside the chamber above the outside or atmospheric pressure. Thus the fresh gases are propelled into the patient's lungs through the endotracheal tube. During expiration, the pressure in the chamber falls again to atmospheric and the stale gases flow out of the lungs escaping to the outside air through a valve. At the same time, the bellows fill with fresh gas in readiness for the next inspiration.

extremely complex equipment designed for prolonged operation in the intensive care unit.

The gases delivered from the ventilator are passed through a humidifier on the way to the patient, since humidification is very important.

Management of ventilator cases

The successful management of ventilator patients requires the highest standards of nursing skill and care. Figure 10.7 summarises some of the most important aspects of this treatment.

Routine tracheostomy regime. The routine care as for other tracheostomy cases is carried out but with one important modification. Most of the patients on ventilators are not breathing at all and can therefore only be disconnected for very short periods

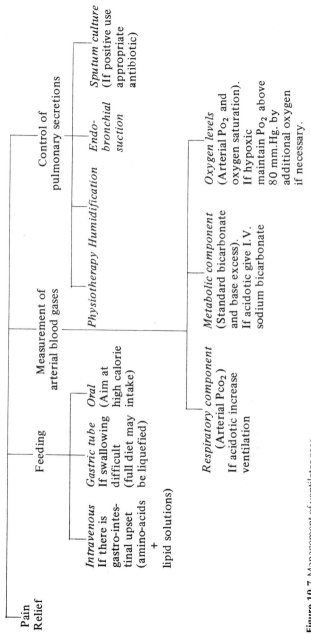

Figure 10.7 Management of ventilator case.

(approximately 1 minute) at a time to permit endobronchial suction. It is usually necessary to perform each period of suction in stages, allowing the patient a few 'breaths' on the machine between each stage.

The management of pain. During ventilator therapy the provision of adequate pain relief can present difficulties, especially in the patient who is unable to communicate. Although the available drugs and techniques of pain relief are many and varied, they are of little value in a situation where the clinician is unable to detect a need for them.

The patient normally reacts to unmodified pain in three possible ways:

a. By making avoidance movements, i.e. attempting to withdraw the injured portion of the body from the stimulus.

b. By responding automatically, e.g. by changes in heart rate and systolic blood pressure.

c. By responding at a cortical level in perceiving the 'painful' stimulus and evaluating it against previous similar experience.

Many of the patients on IPPV are incapable of the first response and indeed may be curarised. Although it has been claimed that the clinician can detect the higher response by complicated electroencephalographic techniques, this is not applicable clinically. Measurements of the autonomic response are as yet the only practicable approach in this difficult situation.

The important thing for the nurse to remember is that an immobile, apparently tranquil, patient on IPPV may be suffering from considerable pain and its relief is an urgent matter. The method and drugs chosen will vary with the individual circumstances but the following list indicates the possibilities:

a. *Parenteral analgesia.* Generally speaking, the intravenous route is to be preferred in this situation since the timing of the peak effect can be more certain and also the relief of pain achieved more quickly. Small incremental doses of say 2 mg morphine sulphate are given intravenously until relief is obtained.

b. *Inhalational analgesia.* It is technically simple with apparatus now available to administer inhalational agents to the patient receiving ventilator therapy, although this method is seldom employed to provide pain relief. A 50% mixture of nitrous oxide in oxygen (Entonox: BOC) is probably the best of the available anaesthetic agents which could be given in this way.

c. Regional blockade. Where it is possible to induce a regional block, complete analgesia of the affected part without any risk of central depression can be achieved. The treatment can be repeated at intervals or maintained continuously as in the case of an epidural block.

Recording of vital functions. In addition to the regular recording of blood pressure, pulse rate and temperature, it is very important that the nurse, under the direction of the anaesthetist, should closely observe and record certain aspects of the ventilator's performance during treatment (Fig. 10.8). For each patient under treatment an ideal pattern of ventilation will have been chosen with regard to frequency of respiration, airway pressure (i.e. the pressure at the patient's mouth during each respiratory cycle of the machine) and the volume of gas being delivered to the patient's lungs (Fig. 10.9). Most respiratory units have a chart on which these events, together with other relevant data, are recorded. The nurse is also trained to listen with a stethoscope over both lungs, at intervals, to make sure that the gases are entering the lungs and not being prevented from doing so by secretions in the upper airway or an obstructed tracheostomy tube.

During the intervals when the patient is disconnected from the ventilator to assess his ability to breathe spontaneously the nurse may be asked to make measurements of the tidal volume as well as the frequency of respiration. For this purpose a spirometer such as the Wright's model can be employed (Fig. 10.10).

Information about the patient's arterial blood gas levels (oxygen tension, pH, Pco_2 and standard bicarbonate) during intermittent positive pressure ventilation, is usually recorded on the ventilation chart by the anaesthetist and the pattern of ventilation may have to be changed at intervals to levels as near normal as possible (Table 10.1 on p. 118). The maintenance of electrolyte and water balance can be difficult in such cases and it is of the first importance to keep *accurate* records on a suitable *Input-Output* Chart.

Monitoring. It must be apparent that the type and number of observations to be made by the attending nurse, particularly in ventilator patients, are liable to be very time consuming. In order to permit more frequent measurements to be made and to free the nurse for other important duties use is increasingly being made of monitoring systems and these systems can be designed to record temperature, heart rate, blood pressure and respiratory rate.

Time and date	O_2 Sat. or Po_2	pH	Pco_2	Stand. Bicarb.	Base excess	Buffer base	On ventilator f V_T P	Off ventilator f V_T	Air Entry in lungs Left Right	Remarks

Key
O_2 **saturation (O_2 sat.):** the percentage of haemoglobin saturated with oxygen in the arterial blood.
Po_2: tension of oxygen in arterial blood.
pH: the degree of acidity or alkalinity of the blood in pH units.
Pco_2: the tension of carbon dioxide in the arterial blood.
Standard bicarbonate ⎤
Base excess ⎬ These measurements indicate the efficiency
Buffer base ⎦ of respiration and the body metabolism.
f: respiratory rate.
V_T: tidal volume.
P: the ventilator pressure during ventilation.
Air entry into lungs: + or − in this column indicates the nurse's assessment of the degree of lung inflation using a stethoscope.

Figure 10.8 Ventilation chart.

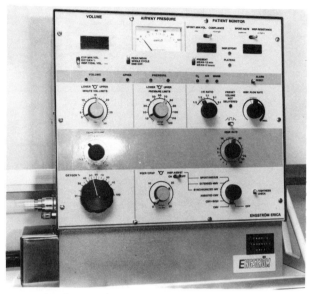

Figure 10.9 Modern lung ventilator (Engstrom Erica). The ventilating volume (minute or tidal) appears as a digital display in the top right hand part of the machine.

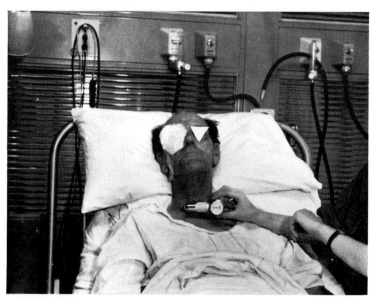

Figure 10.10 The Wright's respirometer being used to measure a patient's minute volume. The instrument is shown attached to a tracheostomy tube.

Table 10.1 Arterial blood gas values: Normal oxygen levels are saturation (Sao_2) over 95% and tension (Pao_2) 90 to 100 mmHg (12–13.5 kPa).

State	pH (Units)	Respiratory Component Pco_2 mmHg (kPa)	Metabolic Component Standard bicarbonate mmol/litre	Base excess mmol/litre
Acidosis	Less than 7.36	More than 44 (5.7)	Less than 22	More than −2.5
Normal	7.36–7.44	36–44 (4.7–5.7)	22–26	±2.5
Alkalosis	More than 7.44	Less than 36 (4.7)	More than 26	More than +2.5

Furthermore the rapid advances in technology which have followed the introduction of small microprocessor based computers incorporating the silicon 'chip' are already spreading to the field of patient care. The data acquired from continuous measurements of the patient's vital functions can now be displayed as trends over a period of time, or further processed to indicate to the clinician and nurse the need for adjustments in therapy, or coupled to alarms giving early warning of potentially dangerous alterations in the patient's condition. The processed data can also be readily stored on discs at the bedside and printed at intervals to provide permanent records for the case-sheet. The new technology is likely to have a great impact on current nursing procedures in intensive care areas and certain to free nurses from the drudgery of charting vital functions, enabling them to apply their skills more directly to the nursing of the patient (Fig. 10.11).

The control of infection. The operation of tracheostomy has been described as potentially lethal in that it opens up a direct route for infection to enter the patient's lungs. In addition, all the patients in an intensive care unit are severely ill and prone intercurrent infection and it is therefore of the utmost importance to minimise the risk of cross-infection from one patient to the other and to isolate any cases of known infection by barrier nursing. Bed-stations should be at least 12 to 14 feet apart since this measure alone greatly reduces the risk of cross-infection. To facilitate isolation of infected cases cubicles are essential, preferably with separate entrances and exits.

A further measure which is of considerable assistance is to ventilate intensive care units, in the same manner as operating theatres, with filtered air, from a positive pressure plenum system. Additional filters can be fitted to suction pumps and ventilator

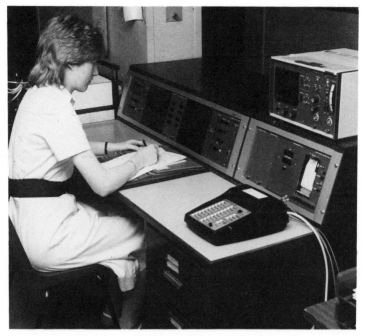

Figure 10.11 Intensive care nursing station showing control buttons for selection of data and paper strips and magnetic tape for recording.

air-pumps to further safeguard the patients. All staff working in the unit should observe the accepted rules governing dress and conduct pertaining in operating theatres.

General care and physiotherapy. These patients must receive particular attention to pressure areas, oral hygiene, eyes and nose. The use of a 'ripple-mattress' greatly reduces the chance of bedsores developing. Many will have indwelling urinary catheters on continuous drainage and intravenous infusions which need constant attention. Passive maintenance exercises to the limbs, percussion of the chest wall and postural drainage are carried out regularly and the physiotherapist has an important function in the treatment of these patients. The dietitian's advice on nutritional problems can be invaluable and hasten the recovery process.

Nurse-patient relationship. Many patients on IPPV are fully conscious but, like all patients with tracheostomies they cannot make their wants known to the nurse or doctor in the usual way. They often become acutely depressed and lose their will to fight, despite continuing physical improvement. The presence of an understanding and cheerful nurse can go a long way towards mitigating what is, for most, a strange and terrifying experience. Some may be able to write their requests and should always have a pad of paper and pencil at hand, but for others it is necessary to provide a simple alphabetical chart with large letters on which the patient can spell out message by pointing with a finger. Great patience is required at this stage and the busy nurse must be prepared to spend a lot of her time in encouraging the patient and keeping up morale.

The unconscious patient

In addition to the measurements already described for the observation and care of respiratory problems certain additional steps must be taken when patient is unconscious.

A varying proportion of the patients in the intensive care area are unconscious. A number of them may have head injuries alone or along with other injuries. Recording the level or degree of unconsciousness is an important and difficult part of the nurse's duties. Accurate observations, recorded frequently by the nurse, can be invaluable in deciding whether an improvement or deterioration is taking place in the patient's condition. There are different levels of consciousness and these may be classified. One such classification is given in Table 10.2.

Table 10.2 Level of consciousness

Stage 1	Stage 2	Stage 3	Stage 4
Patient can answer simple questions	Patient can obey simple commands	Patient reacts only to painful stimuli	Patient fully unconscious — does not react to any stimulus

The vitally important task of monitoring the condition of these patients can be much assisted if a standard method of recording any changes is adopted. One such chart, developed in the Institute of Neurological Sciences at Glasgow, is illustrated in Figure 10.12. The nurse regularly charts the 'best response' so far as eye-opening, speech and movement are concerned and the clinician can see at a glance how the patient's neurological status is changing, if at all.

INSTITUTE OF NEUROLOGICAL SCIENCES, GLASGOW
OBSERVATION CHART

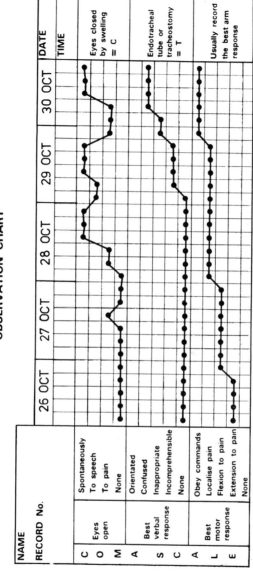

Figure 10.12 The Glasgow coma scale showing observations on a patient over a 5-day period.

Other observation helpful in assessing these patients are rate, depth and character of respiration, rate and volume of pulse, arterial pressure and central venous pressure. In certain neurosurgical cases intracranial pressure changes can be measured directly by means of a cannula inserted through a burr-hole in the skull into the ventricle but this of course carries an added risk of introducing infection.

Acute poisoning

Death from poisoning now rivals that from road accidents in this country. About two-thirds of these deaths are suicidal with the number of females exceeding that of males. Accidental deaths from poisoning are almost exclusively confined to children under 10 years of age.

Of those patients who reach hospital alive, some 10% require the full facilities of an intensive care unit if they are to survive. Following the initial resuscitation and gastric lavage where indicated, the most important aspect of treatment is to maintain a clear airway and support respiration if this is depressed. General supportive measures may also be directed to support depressed cardiovascular function and in some patients to rewarm from a hypothermic state. The techniques already described are therefore applicable in these gravely ill patients and if applied vigorously are usually sufficient to ensure ultimate recovery. In certain instances, however, additional treatment is also aimed at increasing the rate of elimination of the ingested poison from the body and it is appropriate to outline these techniques here, since in many hospitals they are used in the Respiratory Intensive Care Unit as well as the Renal Unit.

Forced diuresis

Forced diuresis is the most commonly employed method to increased the rate of excretion of a drug from the body. It is of most value when a long acting barbiturate such as sodium phenobarbitone has been taken by the patient. Briefly the aim is to increase the urine flow so as to 'wash out' the drug and this process is made more efficient if the urine is kept alkaline. Since it is possible to overload the patient with fluids given in large quantities intravenously it is wise to make regular measurements of central venous pressure during treatment in addition to auscultating the lungs for signs of excessive moisture.

A suitable regime for forced diuresis is as follows:

1. Establish closed urinary drainage; this is an essential preliminary to facilitate the measurement of urine flow at hourly intervals.

2. Establish an intravenous infusion; this is best done by setting up a caval cannula as for central venous pressure measurement. These measurements should be made regularly during the forced diuresis. The infusion is normally begun with 1 litre of normal saline in the first hour followed by 500 ml of 5% dextrose solution in the second hour.

3. An intravenous diuretic such as frusemide (Lasix) is given in repeated doses to maintain a satisfactory urine flow. The fluid input should not be allowed to exceed the output by more than 1 litre and indeed less if there is any sign of circulatory embarassment.

4. If the diuresis is adequate then the intravenous infusion is continued in the following way:

a. 500 ml 5% dextrose in water plus 50 mmol sodium bicarbonate.

b. 500 ml 5% dextrose in water plus 24 mmol potassium chloride.

c. 500 ml normal saline.

Those three solutions are rotated and given at the rate of 500 ml per hour for the duration of treatment. The sodium bicarbonate is given to maintain an alkaline state and the potassium supplement to replace potassium lost in the urine during the diuresis.

Peritoneal dialysis

This technique is occasionally employed as an adjunct to forced diuresis or where haemodialysis is impracticable. Under aseptic conditions a catheter is inserted below the umbilicus under local analgesia. The peritoneal cavity is then lavaged with a dialysing solution containing antibiotic. Figure 10.13 shows the arrangement of the apparatus attached to the catheter. The aim is to use the peritoneum as a dialysing membrane and thus expedite removal of the ingested drug from the body. Usually 1 litre of solution is run in over about 20 minutes. The solution is then allowed to remain for about 20 minutes before being drained off. This cycle is repeated hourly for the duration of treatment.

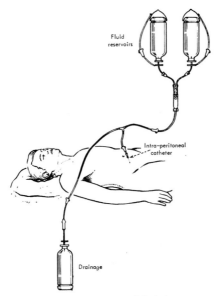

Figure 10.13 Apparatus in use during peritoneal dialysis.

Haemodialysis

The most severely poisoned patients may require haemodialysis. Here the patient's blood is circulated through an artificial kidney machine, some of the drug removed from the blood and the blood returned to the patient. For details of this technique the nurse should study appropriate text-books on the method.

Haemoperfusion

Recently this new technique has been introduced into clinical practice. The patient's blood is allowed to perfuse through a container of activated charcoal which adsorbs the drug. The apparatus is cheap, compact and effective.

It cannot be emphasised too strongly that, while these methods may assist the patient's recovery, survival depends on vigorous application of the general supportive measures already described, in particular those directed towards the support of respiratory function.

Expired air resuscitation or
   mouth-to-mouth
   breathing
External cardiac massage or
   compression

11

Resuscitation

EXPIRED AIR RESUSCITATION OR
MOUTH-TO-MOUTH BREATHING

History

Probably the first written account of this ancient technique is to be found in the Old Testament in the Second Book of Kings. There a description is given of the 'resuscitation' of a young boy by the prophet Elisha and for many hundreds of years the method was known as 'Elisha breathing'. In 1954 Elam and his colleagues demonstrated that expired air resuscitation was more effective than the other standard methods of artificial respiration, e.g. Holger-Nielson and Schafer methods. In 1958 Safar described an airway he designed to make the method easier to perform and in 1960 the Brook airway was first produced.

Table 11.1 Constituents of air samples (approximate values).

Gas	Atmospheric air %	Alveolar air %	Expired air %
Oxygen	21	14.5	14–18
Carbon dioxide	0.04	5.5	4.5
Nitrogen and water vapour	79	80	79

It will be seen from Table 11.1 that atmospheric air contains about 21% oxygen and minimal carbon dioxide. Provided there is an adequate amount of air propelled into the depths of the lungs by the bellows action of the chest and diaphragm and a clear airway, the blood flowing through the lungs in the capillaries will be sufficiently oxygenated (the haemoglobin will be at least 95% saturated with oxygen). In addition, the carbon dioxide carried to the lungs from the tissues will be effectively removed and vented to the atmosphere.

This process of normal ventilation can, of course, be substituted fairly effectively in patients with respiratory arrest by using an apparatus like the Ambu resuscitator to ventilate the lungs with air (atmosphere air resuscitation). Provided the operator compresses the bag often enough and with an adequate depth of stroke and maintains a clear airway, the patient will come to no harm.

It is less easy to understand how the stale expired air of the 'donor' can be adequate to resuscitate a patient. From Table 11.1 it can be seen that expired air contains 14–18% oxygen and 4.5% carbon dioxide. This is more oxygen and less carbon dioxide than is contained in alveolar air from the depths of the lungs, since the latter is mixed with the unused atmospheric air in the air passages on expiration (dead space air). Expired air has been shown to be sufficient to maintain life in volunteers whose respiratory muscles have been temporarily paralysed with curare. The victim's arterial blood contains an adequate quantity of oxygen (the haemoglobin will be about 80% saturated with oxygen) and the carbon dioxide level is reasonably low over long periods of time, e.g. 40 minutes.

During expired air resuscitation the donor uses his own lungs and diaphragm to inflate the victim's lungs. In this way an adequate tidal volume can be maintained.

Technique of mouth-to-mouth breathing

This is best learned on one of the model patients now available, e.g. the Ambu manikin or 'Resuscianne'. All nursing personnel should receive a course of instruction and demonstration, and practise the method for themselves. The correct use of the Safar and Brook airways (Fig. 11.1) which facilitate the technique can be learned at the same time and also the use of the bellows resuscitator for atmospheric air resuscitation (Fig. 11.2).

The following points must be observed:
1. Place the victim on his back if possible.

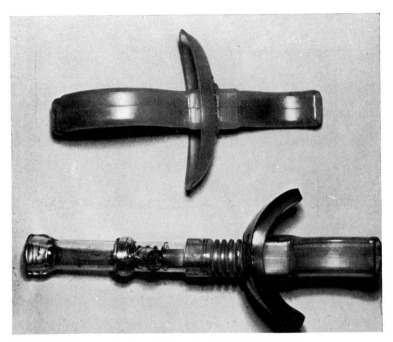

Figure 11.1 Above the Safar and below the Brook airways.

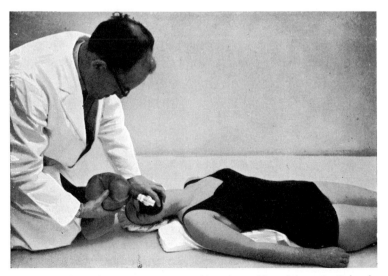

Figure 11.2 The Ambu resuscitator in use. Note the position of the patient's head.

2. Secure a clear airway by posturing the head, removing mucus from the mouth and supporting the lower jaw with the right hand to keep the tongue forward (Fig. 11.3A and B).

3. Apply your mouth to the victim's, making a good seal to prevent leakage of air. In the adult, the nostrils must also be pinched with the fingers of the left hand. In the child, the donor's mouth covers the victim's nostrils and mouth.

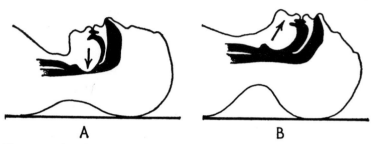

A   **B**

Figure 11.3 These figures demonstrate the correct positioning of the head and jaw during anaesthesia and mouth-to-mouth breathing to ensure a clear airway. In A the head is slightly flexed, the jaw is unsupported and the tongue has fallen back obstructing the upper airway. In B the head has been extended, the jaw pulled forward taking the tongue with it and clearing the airway.

4. Blow until you see the chest rise, removing your mouth to permit expiration. If the stomach fills with air then gentle pressure over it will empty it. The head must then be correctly positioned to improve the airway and prevent a recurrence. If regurgitation of stomach contents takes place the airway must be again cleared before continuing with the resuscitation.

5. Repeat the inflation of the chest 10–20 times/minute.

6. Continue until the patient is breathing adequately for himself or further help and equipment arrive.

7. If the jaw muscles are in spasm and the mouth cannot be opened then the 'mouth to nose' route may be employed after the usual posturing of the head. The latter technique is, in fact, the method preferred by some experts in all cases.

Disadvantages of mouth-to-mouth breathing

There is only *one* apparent *disadvantage* and that is the natural reluctance of the donor to carry out a manoeuvre requiring such intimate contact with the victim. The risk of infection is minimal but in any case such a risk must be weighed against the reward of a successful resuscitation.

Advantages of mouth-to-mouth breathing

The advantages of the method are self-evident.

1. No complicated apparatus is required.

2. The technique is easy to learn and superior to all other methods of artificial respiration.

3. The method is immediately available when most needed, e.g. at the scene of a drowning accident, electrocution in the home, etc.

The method is made easier if a Safar or Brook airway is available but on no account must mouth-to-mouth breathing be delayed when these airways are not immediately available. The nurse has her own 'apparatus' in the form of lungs, mouth and hands.

EXTERNAL CARDIAC MASSAGE OR COMPRESSION

The technique is very simple and can easily be learned. Essentially it comprises intermittent compression of the heart between the mobile sternum in front and the thoracic vertebrae behind (Fig. 11.4). By virtue of the valvular arrangement of the heart, blood is expelled into the aorta and the pulmonary arteries following each compression (artificial systole). On releasing the sternum the heart

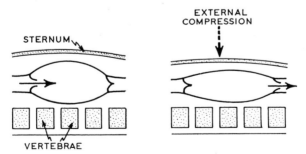

Figure 11.4 This figure shows how the technique of external cardiac massage works. When pressure is applied to the sternum the blood is driven from the heart into the circulation. On release of sternal pressure the heart refills with venous blood in readiness for the next stroke.

fills with blood again (artificial diastole) from the great veins (inferior and superior venae cavae) and the pulmonary veins. The heart is compressed in a cephalad (head-wards) direction and not sideways, this latter movement being prevented by the firm attachment of the pericardium.

The following are the simple steps which make up the manoeuvre:

1. Note the time and clear the airway. Assist ventilation if the patient is not breathing, either by the mouth-to-mouth method or with a resuscitator if one is available.

2. Place the patient on his back on a firm surface, e.g. the floor, or insert fracture boards if in bed. A soft bed prevents effective massage.

3. Place one hand palm down over the lower third of the sternum.

4. The heel of the other hand is now used on top of the lower hand to compress the chest wall intermittently.

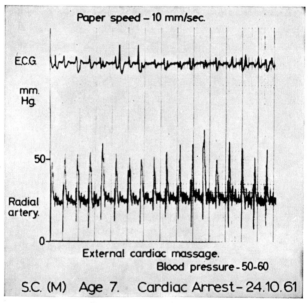

Figure 11.5 Electrocardiograms taken during cardiac massage. The upper tracings are of the e.c.g. and the lower tracings of the blood pressure in the radial artery. The blood pressure is maintained at 50–60 mm Hg (6.5–7.8 kPa) by external cardiac massage.

5. Repeat this sternal compression 60–80 times/minute.

6. In children it is sufficient to compress the sternum with the fingers of one hand only, to avoid undue force and damage to the chest-wall.

7. External cardiac massage is futile unless spontaneous respiration is present and adequate, or alternatively assisted ventilation is simultaneously performed.

The blood which this procedure circulates *must* be oxygenated in the lungs to be of value. A ratio of four sternal compressions to one ventilation of the lungs is recommended.

On the rare occasion when the nurse is single-handed both assistance to ventilation and external cardiac massage can be performed at the one time.

During this emergency someone other than the nurse performing the resuscitation must send for the anaesthetist and/or surgeon in

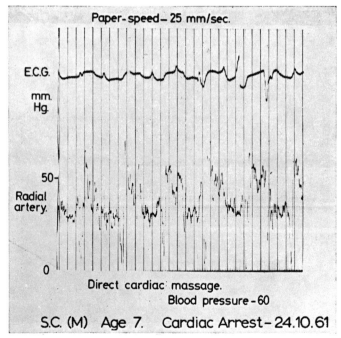

Figure 11.6 The chest has now been opened and direct cardiac massage started. The blood pressure is about 60 mm Hg. (7.8 kPa)

charge of the patient. They may decide to continue with the method or may institute direct cardiac massage after a thoractomy. An e.c.g. will determine whether the heart is arrested in asystole or ventricular fibrillation (Figs 11.5–11.7). If the latter, then electrical defibrillation will be required either externally or directly on the heart itself.

Signs of successful massage

1. An immediate improvement in the patient's colour.
2. Palpable carotid pulses — in time with each sternal compression.
3. Contraction of the pupils.

The resuscitation must continue until these signs of success are present and adequate spontaneous cardiac action and respiration return or until the doctor indicates that hope is abandoned.

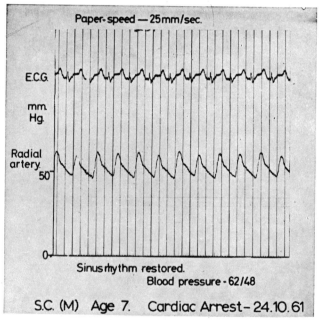

Figure 11.7 Following the cardiac massage and electrical defibrillation of the heart, normal sinus rhythm can be seen on the e.c.g. The blood pressure is 62/48 mm Hg.

Causes of unsuccessful massage

There are two causes of unsuccessful massage:

1. *Inadequate ventilation.* This results in poor oxygenation of the blood returning to the heart and going to the brain.

2. *Ineffective massage.* Commonly ineffective massage is caused by the subject lying on a soft surface, but occasionally it is unavoidable in thick-chested or obese individuals. Direct massage is more effective in the latter case.

12

Anaesthetic machines and other apparatus

Although the early anaesthetics were given with the simplest of apparatus (Fig. 12.1), the modern anaesthetist uses what are to many people large, shiny and complicated machines. While at first sight these machines are indeed complicated they are, in fact, composed of five simple systems (Fig. 12.2).

1. A supply of compressed gases.
2. A method of reducing these gases to workable pressure.
3. A method of releasing and metering the gases.
4. A method of vaporising volatile anaesthetic agents.
5. A means of delivering the gases and vapours to the patient.

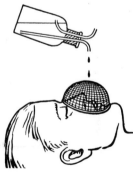

Figure 12.1 Wire frame mask covered with gauze on which agent is dropped.

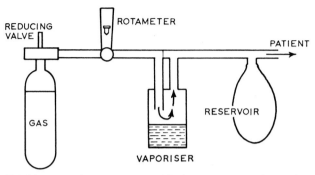

Figure 12.2 Diagrammatic representation of the five components of a simple anaesthetic apparatus.

The supply of gases

This may take one of two forms. On most machines there is provision for two cylinders of nitrous oxide, two of oxygen, one of carbon dioxide and one of cyclopropane. These cylinders may be used as the main supply of gases and the machine in this case is fairly mobile. It is customary to use one nitrous oxide cylinder and one oxygen cylinder at any one time, keeping the other tightly closed and in reserve. In hospitals where considerable quantities of these gases are used, it is more economical to buy them in large cylinders which are stored at a convenient place some distance from the theatre and the gases are then piped to the theatres, connection being made between the end of the pipeline and the anaesthetic machine. Oxygen may be stored in liquid form and this is a further saving in cost. Even where the pipeline system is employed, however, at least one cylinder of each gas should be kept on the machine as a reserve in case of failure of the pipeline supply.

The cylinders are readily identifiable, each being painted in a distinctive colour—oxygen being black with white shoulders, nitrous oxide blue, cyclopropane orange and carbon dioxide grey. In addition the name of the gas is printed on the cylinder as is the chemical symbol. A further safeguard against connecting a cylinder to the wrong reducing valve is that in the head of the cylinder beside the port, out of which the gas flows, two small holes are drilled in positions specified for each gas (Fig. 12.3). These match two pins on the reducing valve.

In addition to identifying the cylinders containing a particular gas, it is important to know how much of the gas each cylinder

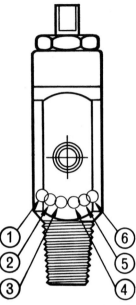

Figure 12.3 This diagram shows how the holes on the cylinder neck are drilled on an arc. Only two holes are found on each cylinder e.g.: 2 & 5 on oxygen cylinders 3 & 5 on nitrous oxide cylinders 3 & 6 on cyclopropane cylinders.

contains. In the case of oxygen, the reducing valve connected to the cylinder has attached to it a pressure gauge and the contents of the cylinder can be measured by estimating the pressure. A full cylinder contains gas at a pressure of approximately 2000 lb/sq in and as the volume of gas in the cylinder falls the pressure is proportionally reduced. A device is available which gives visual and audible warning when the oxygen cylinder is empty. Nitrous oxide and carbon dioxide are however stored as liquids and the pressure above the liquid remains the same until very little liquid remains in the cylinder (Fig. 12.4). Because of this a pressure gauge would inform the anaesthetist only at this stage. This indication is however better than none and, in some modern anaesthetic machines, the pressure gauge is again being incorporated in the reducing valve for use with nitrous oxide. The normal method of ascertaining how much nitrous oxide remains in the cylinder, however, is to weigh the cylinder and by subtracting the tare weight of the cylinder, which is embossed on the neck, one can determine how much nitrous oxide is left in the cylinder (200 gallons of nitrous oxide weigh 60 oz or 100 litres nitrous oxide weigh 0.8 kg).

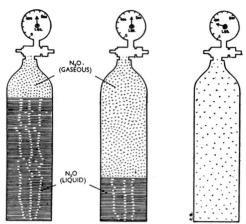

Figure 12.4 Pressure of N_2O as recorded by gauge remains constant until very little liquid remains in the cylinder.

Clip-on labels are provided which attach to the reducing valve showing the words 'full', 'in use' or 'empty'. When a cylinder becomes empty it should preferably be removed at once and be replaced with a full cylinder, failing which an 'empty' label should be placed on the reducing valve. If this is not possible, it is wise to disconnect the reducing valve from the cylinder as a reminder that this cylinder must be replaced at the first opportunity.

The nurse should make a point of finding out where full cylinders of anaesthetic gases are kept. A full cylinder normally has a red cellophane wrapper covering the outlet port and if this is not in place the cylinder should be treated as empty until proved otherwise.

Reducing valves

Apart from cyclopropane the pressures of the gases in the cylinders vary from 700 to 2000 lb/sq in (48.3×10^5 to 138×10^6 Pa). Such pressures are, of course, not manageable when metering the gases through the anaesthetic machine and they must be reduced to workable levels. The valve in common use in this country is called an Adams' valve (Fig. 12.5). Each valve bears colours similar to the cylinder for which it is intended and is also labelled with the name of the appropriate gas. It bears pins which will fit into the holes drilled in the head of the cylinder, fitting only the corresponding cylinder.

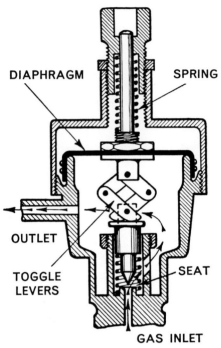

DIAPHRAGM   **SPRING**

OUTLET

TOGGLE   **SEAT**
LEVERS

GAS INLET

Figure 12.5 Working principle of Adams' valve.

The nitrous oxide and carbon dioxide valves in addition have fluting on them which presents a larger surface for absorption of heat since the nitrous oxide and carbon dioxide are changing state and therefore absorbing heat. Without the fluting the reducing valve might freeze and cease to function.

Flow meters

The flow meters in common use are known as Rotameters. They consist of tapered glass tubes in which spin aluminium bobbins (Fig. 12.6). The spinning bobbin is not in contact with the side of the tube and is therefore unlikely to stick. This avoids false readings of gas flow. The gas flow is indicated by the figure on the rotameter opposite the top of the bobbin.

Vaporisers

These may be divided into two types. The simple vaporiser (Fig. 12.7) is suitable for vaporisation of trichloroethylene and ether

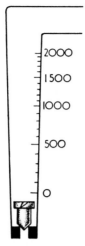

Figure 12.6 The Rotameter. As gas enters at the lower end the spinning bobbin rises in proportion to the flow of gas.

where the exact concentration of the vapour is not critical. A level at the side of the bottle directs an increasing amount of the gas into the bottle and when the plunger is depressed the stream of gases coming up the J tube is directed on to or indeed through the fluid in

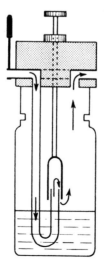

Figure 12.7 A simple vaporiser—the Boyle's bottle. The arrows indicate the direction of gas flow.

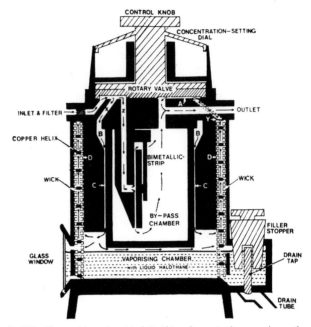

Figure 12.8 The Fluotec Vaporiser Mark 3. This schematic diagram shows the construction of the vaporiser. The concentration-setting dial is in an 'on' position. A = vapour control chamber; B = annular expansion chamber; C = long annular throat; D = spiral outlet channel of vaporising chamber; X = inlet to vaporising chamber; Y = outlet from vaporising chamber; Z = inlet to bypass chamber. (From Paterson GM, Hulands G H, Nunn J F 1969 British Journal of Anaesthesia 41 : 109)

the bottle. When using more powerful drugs such as halothane, vaporisers which compensate for changes in temperature and other factors are employed. One of these is the Fluotec (Fig. 12.8) which delivers halothane in increments of 0.5%.

Delivery of the gases and vapours to the patient

This may be achieved by using a *Magill attachment* (Fig. 12.9) consisting of a corrugated rubber tube, a reservoir bag, and a spill valve. The reservoir is necessary since the flow of gas from the machine is continuous during all phases of respiration whereas the patient's demand for these gases is only during inspiration. At the patient's end of the tube is placed the valve through which excess gas may pass and connection may be made with a mask which is placed over the patient's face.

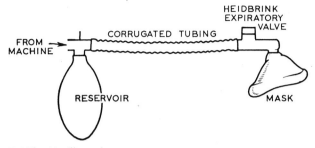

Figure 12.9 The Magill attachment.

A non-return or non-rebreathing valve (Fig. 12.10) may be used instead of the conventional Heidbrink valve. In this case during expiration all the expired gas passes to the atmosphere and re-breathing of carbon dioxide is minimal. The T-piece circuit (Fig. 12.11) introduced by Ayre is used in children when the resistance to expiration offered by valves is harmful to the child,

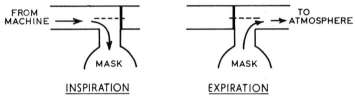

Figure 12.10 A non-return valve. During inspiration the valve slides across and permits the patient to breathe gases from the machine. On expiration the valve cuts off the supply of gases from the machine and allows the expired gas from the patient to pass to the atmosphere.

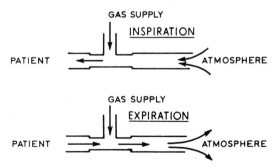

Figure 12.11 The T-piece principle. As there are no valves, resistance is minimal and, by adjusting the flow of gases and the length of the expiratory limb to the atmosphere, the degree of rebreathing can be controlled.

particularly if spontaneous respiration is to occur for a prolonged period. The open limb of the T-piece conveys expired gas to the atmosphere and acts as a reservoir.

A *closed circuit* may also be used. Using such a system it is possible to pass the patient's expiration to the machine and back again, directing the expired gases through soda-lime to absorb the carbon dioxide which is given off and adding oxygen as the gas is passed back to the patient (Fig. 12.12).

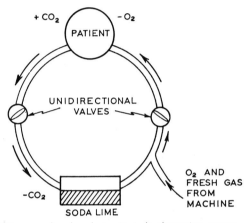

Figure 12.12 Diagram of a closed circuit circle absorption system.

The removal of exhaust gases is now assuming increased importance. Although the theatre atmosphere may only contain very low concentrations of gas or vapour repeated exposures to these may be harmful to theatre personnel. It is now possible, where a closed circuit is not being used, to lead the waste gases outside the theatre or to an adsorption canister.

Intermittent flow machines

Most anaesthetic machines are based on the continuous flow principle, that is, the fresh gas flows to the circuit at a constant rate throughout all phases of breathing, the excess during expiration being held in a reservoir. Other systems such as the Walton apparatus for dental anaesthesia and the Entonox analgesia apparatus supply gases to the patient only in response to the patient's respiratory effort (Fig. 12.13). It is essential to ensure a gas-tight fit

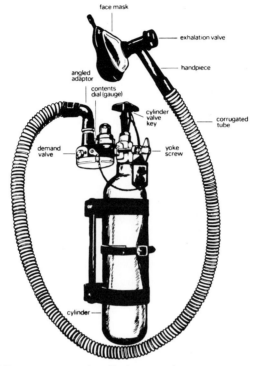

Figure 12.13 Entonox apparatus for self-administered 50 per cent nitrous oxide in oxygen. The gas leaves the cylinder only when the patient makes an inspiratory effort.

between the patient's face and the mask or the system will not function satisfactorily.

The care and maintenance of anaesthetic machines

The responsibility for looking after anaesthetic machines varies from hospital to hospital and, in many theatres, the technician will do what is required. It is valuable, however, for a nurse to know what to do and what to leave alone.

After use the shelves on the machine should be cleared and cleaned, usually with soap and water. Do not throw buckets full of water over the machine — this is both unnecessary and harmful. The rubber tubing should be detached, complete with metal connections when present, washed in warm soapy water, rinsed and hung up to dry. Any volatile anaesthetic left in the simple vaporisers should be discarded unless instructions are given to the contrary. Do not, on your own initiative, return the contents to stock bottles. If gas cylinders are in use they should be turned off with the key provided. Empty cylinders should be replaced with full ones. Pipeline connections should be disconnected and suction bottles emptied and cleaned.

When setting up theatre for use, the tubing should be returned to the machine and a supply of facemasks made available. The pipeline connections should be firmly joined together—the ends are coloured to indicate which gas they are for and the couplings are non-interchangeable. Where soda-lime is used regularly it should be replaced daily or a fresh supply laid out ready for use.

It is seldom that these simple duties should be exceeded although local arrangements may determine what part the anaesthetist, technician and theatre staff play in attending to the anaesthetic machine. These machines have many removable parts and a curious nurse may misguidedly take them to pieces 'to clean them'. DON'T — lest like a little boy and his watch, you find when you have put it together again you have enough pieces left over to make another one!

Sterilisation of machines

While, in most instances, the tubing on the machines is merely washed, rinsed and dried as described, where a patient with a serious respiratory infection has been anaesthetised more stringent measures are employed.

The tubing may be autoclaved after thorough washing and will withstand this treatment several times. More thorough sterilisation is achieved by treating, in a closed circuit, anaesthetic machines and ventilators, with a mixture of ethylene oxide and carbon dioxide ('Carboxide').

SUCTION APPARATUS

In anaesthetic practice, the immediate availability of efficient suction apparatus can be life-saving. Although there are many other surgical uses for this type of equipment, generally speaking the anaesthetist requires more powerful and often portable apparatus for the removal of mucus or vomitus from the stomach or respiratory tract. The low flow suction apparatus used for continuous gastric drainage in the wards is not suitable for anaesthetic purposes. Three types of apparatus are worthy of special mention:

1. Simple portable equipment requiring no power supply.
2. Electrically driven high vacuum suction apparatus.
3. Pipeline suction apparatus powered by compressed gas.

1. Portable suction apparatus

The Ambu foot pump suction apparatus (Fig. 12.14) is a useful emergency aid for the anaesthetist when the situation is such that no power driven apparatus is available. It is adequate for the removal of fluid or mucus of low viscosity and where very large quantities of material are present.

2. Electrical high vacuum suction machines

The Matburn suction apparatus (Fig. 12.15) is a good example of this type. It is capable of producing high vacuum suction for the

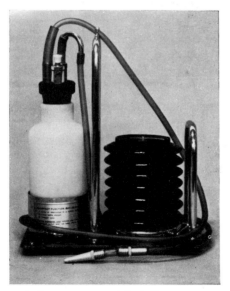

Figure 12.14 The Ambu foot suction pump. The bellows is intermittently compressed by the foot thus creating a vacuum in the reservoir bottle. Aspirated material collects in the bottle.

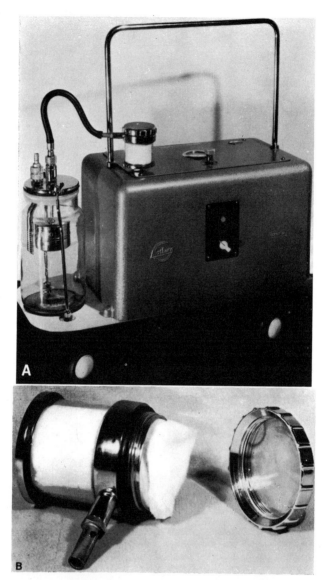

Figure 12.15 The Matburn suction apparatus. A, The dial on the top of the apparatus indicates the negative pressure which may be adjusted by the control knob beside the dial. B, The bacteriological filter which prevents dispersion of infected material into the surrounding air.

removal of viscid material or low vacuum, high flow suction for large quantities of less viscid fluids. The machine is mounted on castors and is therefore manoeuvrable in the anaesthetic room or recovery ward provided an electrical power point is at hand. The motor is sealed and the apparatus is thus safe to use in the presence of oxygen or combustible anaesthetic vapours.

3. Pipeline suction apparatus

Many theatre suites and intensive care units have piped suction along with piped oxygen and nitrous oxide. Figure 12.16 shows a typical apparatus of this type. There are independent vacuum and flow controls so that the correct setting can be obtained for viscid or low viscosity material.

The problem of bacterial contamination

When infected material is aspirated the liquid bubbles in the receiving bottle and forms a fine spray which is sucked through the pump and discharged into the atmosphere. This is obviously highly

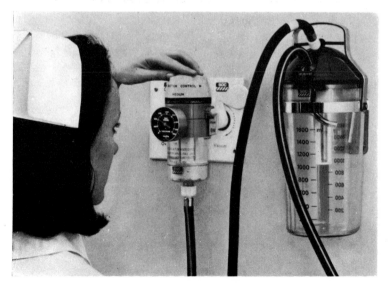

Figure 12.16 Pipeline suction unit. The controls permit independent adjustment of vacuum and flow rate. A bacterial filter is interposed between the collection flask and the vacuum pipeline.

undesirable in a ward where other non-infected patients are being simultaneously treated. Low vacuum apparatus causes less foaming and bubbling and is less of a danger in this respect but some form of filter is desirable in other apparatus.

Reservoir bottles must be emptied with care to prevent nursing and medical staff being infected and should be cleaned and sterilised before further use. The bottle should then be primed with a small quantity of antiseptic solution, e.g. Hibitane or Roccal. The suction tubing at the patient's end of the apparatus should be cleaned and autoclaved before being used on another patient if disposable tubing has not been used.

The nozzle of the suction pipe, when not in use, should be protected from contamination by immersion in a container of antiseptic fluid.

Vacuum and flow control

The need to be able to vary the vacuum and flow controls separately in suction apparatus has already been alluded to. In general, high vacuum should only be used for thick or tenacious fluids, low vacuum with a high flow being preferable for less viscid fluids and for large quantities of non-viscous material. Low vacuum suction is less damaging to the mucosa of the mouth and respiratory tract and also causes less frothing and dissemination of infected material. All apparatus should have a vacuum gauge in a position where the negative pressure applied can be easily read and excessive vacuum thereby avoided.

Assembly and testing of suction apparatus

After the suction apparatus and tubing have been cleaned and sterilised they must be carefully reassembled and left ready for use. If all joints are airtight, when the machine is operated and the nozzle occluded, the maximum vacuum should be obtained and this is shown on the dial. If this is not so, recheck the apparatus for air leaks or enlist the help of an engineer.

ELECTRICAL DEFIBRILLATORS

Electrical defibrillators are essential for the treatment of cardiac arrest. The apparatus may be used internally with the electrodes applied directly to the surface of the heart by the operator or externally with the electrodes applied to the chest wall. Two types of machine are in common use, A.C. (alternating current) and D.C. (direct current) defibrillators, and both can be used internally or externally. The D.C. defibrillator is now preferred since this type of current has been shown to be more effective in reversing ventricular fibrillation.

Since the apparatus must be constantly at the ready alongside the cardiac arrest trolley, it must be checked regularly to ensure that it is in perfect order. High voltages are used for electrical defibrillation, particularly for the external procedure, and the operator should wear rubber gloves when holding the electrodes. Figure 12.17 illustrates one model and the large electrodes which are applied to the chest wall can be seen. The large surface area of these electrodes reduces the chance of burning the patient's skin and this risk is further minimised by rubbing the skin with e.c.g. electrode jelly before the procedure.

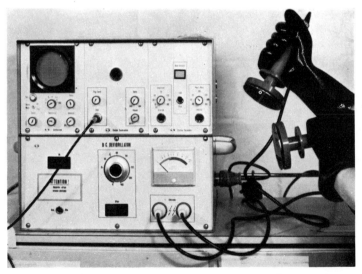

Figure 12.17 An electrical defibrillator with electrodes set up for external use.

J. F. Chisholm, SRD
Dietitian, Glasgow Royal infirmary

Appendix 1

Diets for special cases

During the early part of the patient's stay in the respiratory emergency unit all feeding and fluid administration will probably be by the intravenous route, supervised by the physician in charge. At a later stage a change is normally made to feeding by intragastric tube and subsequently to feeding by mouth when the patient is able to swallow adequately. The nurse may have the responsibility of preparing suitable feeds for these patients and a knowledge of the dietetic problems involved is essential. In a respiratory emergency unit two types of patient are most frequently met with where special feeding is required. One is the patient receiving prolonged ventilator therapy and the other the patient who may or may not be on a ventilator, but has some degree of renal failure.

The detailed diets described below are given to assist the nurse who may have to attend to the special feeding problems of such patients without the help of a trained dietitian.

1. PATIENT ON VENTILATOR: A HIGH PROTEIN, HIGH CALORIE DIET TO BE GIVEN BY INTRA-GASTRIC ROUTE

For a man or woman in normal health and having a sedentary occupation, approximately 2500 calories (10.5 mega-joules) and

2100 calories (8.6 mega-joules) respectively are required. Protein intake should be approximately 70 g and 60 g respectively.*

Any severe injury or major surgical operation leads to tissue destruction and loss; therefore if weight is to be gained and tissue replacement made the diet must supply *more than* the above figures for protein and, where possible, a 'credit balance' of calories as well.

The two diets given below aim at replacement of tissue by giving a protein total of 140 g (i.e. approximately twice normal needs) and 2800 calories (11.8 mega-joules), bearing in mind that since these patients are in bed their calorific requirements are lower than normal.

Even higher calorific intakes can be achieved by giving extra glucose, Gastro-Caloreen (Scientific Hospital Supplies) and Prosparol (Duncan Flockhart, Edinburgh). Gastro-Caloreen is a glucose polymer which dissolves very easily in a small quantity of fluid. It should not cause nausea and vomiting which can be induced by strong glucose solutions of equal concentration. One hundred grams of Gastro-Caloreen provides 400 calories. Prosparol is a fat emulsion containing 50% of a vegetable oil. In 100 ml there are 45 g of fat with a calorific value of 405.

The following are suitable diets for these patients:

In diet A Complan (Glaxo) is used, either alone or with addition of glucose or Gastro-Caloreen. This is only one example of many commercially available preparations for the purpose.

In diet B a variety of foods is used.

A. An intra-gastric feed using Complan (Glaxo) includes all known nutrients in 'ideal' proportions

Quantity for 1 day:
1 lb packet of Complan dissolved in water gives:

Protein (g)	Fat (g)	Carbohydrate (g)
140	74	200
(× 4)	(× 9)	(× 4)
560 cal	666 cal	800 cal
	Total = 2026 calories	

* Department of Health and Social Security 1969. Recommended intakes of nutrients.

If 180 g of glucose or Gastro-Caloreen are added to this feed, the carbohydrate will then be 380 g and calories raised to approximately 2800. Methyl cellulose granules (e.g. Celevac) may also have to be added to prevent diarrhoea.

B. Normal diet liquidised

Quantity for 1 day (figures from McCance RA, Widdowson EM 1967 The composition of foods, 2nd edn. HMSO, London):

	Weight (g)	Protein (g)	Fat (g)	Carbohydrate (g)
Breakfast				
Porridge	150	2.1	1.4	12.3
Milk	150	5.1	5.6	7.2
Egg	60	7.1	7.4	–
Glucose	50	–	–	50.0
Double cream	30	0.5	14.5	0.6
		14.8	28.9	70.1
Lunch				
Meat	120	32.0	20.0	–
Potato	90	1.3	–	17.7
Sieved vegetable	60	–	–	5.0
Milk pudding	200	6.8	7.8	35.0
Milk	500	17.0	18.5	24.0
Fruit juice	100	–	–	10.0
Marmite	1 teasp.			
Methyl cellulose granules	2			
50 mg vitamin C tablet				
		57.1	46.3	91.7
Supper Similar to lunch				
Bedtime				
Milk	200	6.8	7.4	9.6
Skim milk powder	15	5.2	0.1	7.4
Horlicks	10	1.4	0.8	7.1
		13.4	8.3	24.1
Breakfast		14.8	28.9	70.1
Lunch		57.1	46.3	91.7
Supper		57.1	46.3	91.7
Bedtime		13.4	8.3	24.1

Calories = 2848

Many units now find that the most satisfactory way to maintain a patient's nutritional status is by giving a normal diet which has been liquidised either in the diet kitchen or at the ward. As the patient is not required to taste this diet, a complete cooked meal can be put together and either liquidised or sieved so that the final mixture is smooth enough to go down a tube.

2. PATIENT WHO IS HAVING HIGH PROTEIN, HIGH CALORIE DIET BY MOUTH

When the appetite is poor it may be necessary to use high protein supplements, e.g. Casilan (Glaxo), Forceval-Protein (Unigreg), etc. to achieve a high calorie, high protein diet. The main aim in using these supplements is to increase the calorie and protein content of the dish without increasing the bulk or altering the flavour.

Fortified milk mixtures can be used instead of plain milk in drinks, milk puddings, etc. and assure an intake of approximately 50–60 g protein, so that even with very small servings of meat, eggs, etc. one can reasonably expect to reach a total of over 100 g protein per day.

Sample recipes for fortified milk mixtures

		Protein (approx. in g)
(a)	2 pt liquid milk	40
	2 oz full cream dried milk	15
		55
(b)	2 pt liquid milk	40
	2 oz dried skim milk	20
		60

N.B. Ordinary milk should be used for tea and coffee.

Sample menu for day. Soft diet, quantities according to appetite:

Breakfast:	Fruit or fruit juice, with sugar, or fine porridge with milk.
	1 or 2 eggs, scrambled or soft boiled.
	Bread, butter, marmalade.
	Tea or coffee using plain milk, sugar.

Mid-morning:	Drink made with 'fortified milk'. (This can be flavoured with banana, apricot or blackcurrant purée, or Ribena, cocoa, coffee or Crusha milk shake syrup.
Dinner:	Cream soup. Serving of minced meat, fish cream, chicken fricassée or similar dish. Creamed potato. Puréed vegetable. Sweet (high in protein) e.g. caramel custard with cream, milk jelly using fortified milk, or fruit whip with Casilan and cream. Tea using plain milk, sugar.
Tea:	Tea, milk, sugar. (or fortified drink as at mid-morning) Small sandwich if desired, with cream cheese or honey. Piece of light sponge.
Supper:	Similar to dinner. Include sweet wherever possible.
Bedtime:	Fortified milk drink as above.

3. URAEMIC PATIENT

1. In this case it must be remembered that the kidney is unable to excrete the end-products of protein metabolism, i.e. urea, uric acid etc. There is nitrogen retention due to the excretion being impaired and therefore the blood urea level rises. It is important that the minimum of protein be given at this stage.

2. Since fluid is not being lost in the urine, only the 'obligatory loss', i.e. fluid lost through sweating and respiration, may be given. In these patients there is increased production of water from endogenous fat breakdown, and thus the amount allowed is restricted to approximately 500 ml.

3. Endogenous protein breakdown can be decreased by giving high calories from non-protein sources, i.e. fats and carbohydrates. Initially, a high calorie, protein free, electrolyte-free diet should be given. A great advance in this respect was the introduction of Bull's régime, which consisted of 400 g of glucose and 100 g of peanut-oil in 1 litre of water administered by the intra-gastric route as a fine emulsion. This provides a total of 2500 calories (10.5 mega-joules).

Although Bull's diet is seldom used now in the United Kingdom, it may prove useful in overseas countries.

Nowadays there are various proprietary foods available which can be used to provide or supplement a high calorie, electrolyte-free diet. Caloreen (Scientific Hospital Supplies) and Hycal (Beechams) are probably tolerated best. Caloreen is a glucose polymer which is relatively non-sweet to taste. It blends with most foods and will dissolve very easily in a small quantity of fluid. Caloreen, whose calorific value is similar to that of sugar, is very suitable for the nauseated patient. (Gastro-Caloreen is virtually identical with Caloreen but Gastro-Caloreen contains electrolytes and is therefore not always suitable for renal conditions.) Caloreen has been specially prepared as an electrolyte-free substance.

Hycal is a ready-to-drink preparation made from Liquid Glucose B.P.C. that has been demineralised and is supplied in six flavours to give variety. Hycal is supplied in 175 ml bottles, each bottle containing 425 calories.

Sucrose, glucose or other sugars may be used but these tend, in high concentrations, to be rather sweet and may cause nausea and/or diarrhoea.

All these sugars can be given orally or via an intra-gastric drip. The total volume allowed depends on the previous day's output.

In all cases extreme care must be taken to avoid the use of high potassium fruit juices as a base for sugar or glucose since hyper-kalaemia is often present. It is for this reason that both Hycal and Caloreen are so popular since they are practically electrolyte-free. Tea and coffee, particularly instant coffee, should be treated with caution as they both contain potassium.

For patients able to eat, most authorities now advocate a diet consisting mainly of carbohydrate and fat and with a very low protein content, e.g. 10 g.

Sample menu for day

Breakfast:	Fruit or fruit juice with added sugar or glucose. Cereal, e.g. Cornflakes, Rice Krispies. *No porridge.* Double cream if desired. Tea, sugar, lemon if desired. *No milk.*
Mid-morning:	Fruit drink with glucose, e.g. fruit squash.
Dinner:	Vegetable soup, e.g. tomato, celery. Two tablespoon gravy.

	Vegetable, e.g. turnip mashed with butter. *No pulses.*
	Potato—mashed with butter.
	Fruit and sugar, e.g. fruit salad.
	Double cream if desired.
Tea:	One thin slice white bread, butter, jam, honey. Tea, sugar. *No milk.*
Supper:	Vegetable dish, e.g. vegetable hot pot, stuffed tomatoes.
	One thin slice white bread, butter, jam, honey. Tea, sugar. *No milk.*
Bedtime:	Fruit drink with glucose.

4. PATIENT RECOVERING FROM ACUTE RENAL FAILURE

(It is assumed that in this patient the blood urea level is still raised but food is now being given by mouth.)

The same principles apply as in the previous case.

1. Protein intake must still be limited. The example given shows a diet containing approximately 20 g of protein, which can be increased gradually as the blood urea level falls.

2. As before. Calories from non-protein sources should be high to minimise breakdown of body protein.

3. Fluid intake is still measured and depends on urinary output; an amount equivalent to the volume of urine passed is added to the 1 litre obligatory loss already mentioned.

4. Since the kidney is not yet excreting electrolytes efficiently at this stage, the diet may have to be controlled in either sodium or potassium.

Confusion sometimes arises as to the exact quantity of sodium the doctor wishes to employ in a salt-restricted diet. The following table shows the various terms used and the quantities of sodium involved:

Sodium intakes	mmol Na^+/day
Normal free salt, according to choice	60–300
Restricted (no salty foods, no salt added at table)	60–80
Low (no salt used in cooking or at table, salty foods avoided)	40–50

Very low (as above, but with use of salt-free bread and salt-free butter)	15–30
Minimal or ultra low—requires the use of formulae and special foods	less than 15

1 g NaCl = 17 mmol Na$^+$

When the diet is low in protein the sodium content will be at the lower end of the range indicated.

If the potassium content of the diet has to be controlled, fruit juices, fruit and vegetables should be included only in moderate amounts.

At a later stage in the recovery from acute renal failure—the diuretic phase—it may be necessary to increase the electrolytes in the diet or depletion can occur. Great care should be taken and sodium and potassium should be increased only as required.

Sample menu for day:

Breakfast:	Fruit or fruit juice, with added sugar or glucose. Cereal, e.g. Cornflakes, Rice Krispies. *No porridge.* One thin slice white bread, butter, marmalade. Tea, one tablespoon milk, sugar.
Mid-morning:	Fruit drink with glucose, e.g. fruit squash.
Dinner:	Vegetable soup, e.g. tomato, celery. 1 oz meat, fish, chicken, etc. (N.B. rissoles, kedgeree, etc. help to disguise small size of protein servings.) Vegetables, e.g. carrot, cabbage—good helping. *No pulses.* Potato—good helping. Fruit and sugar, e.g. fruit salad, tinned fruit. (Double cream may be given with these.)
Tea:	One thin slice white bread, butter, jam. Tea, one tablespoon milk, sugar.
Supper:	Vegetable dish, e.g. vegetable hot pot, salad, etc. Fruit if liked. One thin slice white bread, butter, jam. Tea, one tablespoon milk, sugar. Shortbread or biscuits made with cornflour or arrowroot only can be used as extras.
Bedtime:	Fruit drink with glucose.

D. Anderson, MCSP
(Teacher's certificates)
*Principal, School of Physiotherapy,
Glasgow Royal Infirmary*

Appendix 2

Notes on physiotherapy for the nurse

These notes are intended for the guidance of nurses who may be asked to deal with certain postoperative complications, and who are without the services of a trained physiotherapist. The highly specialised field of physiotherapy following thoracic surgery is excluded from this simplified appendix.

The postoperative complications most likely to require the attention of a physiotherapist are pulmonary and vascular in origin. They may follow any operation no matter what type of anaesthetic is used, but are more liable to occur after thoracic and abdominal surgery, particularly in elderly patients or in those already suffering from some pulmonary or vascular disease, e.g. chronic bronchitis.

PULMONARY COMPLICATIONS

In the immediate postoperative period the patient's pulmonary ventilation is reduced for many reasons (Ch 9). These include:

1. Depression of the cough reflex.
2. Excessive secretion of sticky mucus.
3. Pain and muscle spasm due to the incision, particularly in the case of abdominal surgery.
4. Mild postoperative shock.

It is essential that the patient be made to ventilate his lungs fully, and to cough up the accumulating secretions thus reducing the possibility of a blockage in a bronchus or bronchiole with consequent collapse of part or, in some cases, all of the lung.

VASCULAR COMPLICATIONS

Venous thrombosis sometimes follows operation and, as yet, the exact mechanism is not understood. The thrombus usually appears in a vein of the lower limb and the following factors are known to predispose to this complication:

1. An increased tendency for the blood to clot following operation, particularly after lower abdominal incisions.
2. Considerable slowing of the circulation due to the patient lying flat in bed and remaining very still after operation.
3. Minor damage to the walls of veins because the tone of muscles which usually protects the veins is considerably reduced during anaesthesia and surgery.

If a thrombus forms there is danger that a small portion (embolus) will break off and lodge in the lungs. If such a pulmonary embolus is large it may block the pulmonary artery, and death quickly follows.

The object of physiotherapy is to *prevent* these complications from occurring.

It is unrealistic to expect a patient in the immediate postoperative phase to co-operate unless the reason for the various procedures is understood, so that it is necessary to visit the patient preoperatively.

PREOPERATIVE STAGE

1. Explain to the patient the need for postoperative treatment.
2. Teach the patient breathing exercises.
3. Teach the patient how to cough adequately.
4. Teach the patient simple leg and foot movements.

Explanation

Some discretion may be necessary to avoid alarming the patient, but in most cases, it is helpful to explain the reason for the various physiotherapeutic procedures. If in doubt, consult the doctor.

Breathing exercises

Two simple breathing exercises should be taught:

a. *Diaphragmatic breathing.* Always begin with expiration. Ask the patient to breathe out, sinking the upper chest. At the end of expiration, tighten the abdominal muscles gently. Relax the tightened abdominal muscles and breathe in, filling the lower part of the lungs. The patient's head should be supported and the arms and shoulder girdle relaxed. On breathing in, the upper chest should remain still and the abdomen swell outwards. A firm hand placed on the abdomen between the angle of the ribs will indicate to the patient where the movement should occur.

A patient with an abdominal incision may be very reluctant to practise diaphragmatic breathing because it produces tension on the incision and, in these cases, it may be delayed for 2 or 3 days, practising lateral costal breathing in the meantime.

b. *Lateral costal breathing.* A similar procedure is adopted. The patient breathes out, sinking the upper chest, and tightening the abdominal muscles. In this case the physiotherapist's hands are placed on either side of the rib cage, giving firm pressure, and encouraging the patient to expand the ribs sideways.

These breathing exercises should be practised assiduously until the patient becomes proficient.

Coughing

The patient should be taught how to produce a deep 'abdominal' cough, and warned against the shallow, irritating 'throat' cough which is ineffective in removing sputum.

Effective coughing is brought about by a short, sharp expiration with strong contractions of the diaphragm.

In patients with an abdominal incision this method of coughing produces some strain on the wound which may prevent the patient from coughing adequately. This tendency will be reduced if the patient is shown how to support the incision with both hands.

Leg and foot exercises

The extent and scope of these exercises will depend on the condition of the patient, e.g. strong leg exercises will be contraindicated in many abdominal operations. The following simple exercises may be used in all conditions and, in conjunction with the breathing exercises already described, will help to maintain the circulation in the legs, and so reduce the chances of thrombus formation.

a. Push toes of both feet towards the end of bed. Relax. Pull toes up to chin. Relax.

b. Circle both ankles, first one way and then the other. Repeat three times and relax.

c. Bend each knee alternately, sliding foot up bed. Relax.

d. Thrust both feet towards end of bed bracing all leg muscles. Relax.

Note that the movements should be performed fairly slowly and with strong muscle contractions, and that each movement should be followed by a short period of complete relaxation. In addition, the patient should be warned of the danger of lying completely still in bed after operation.

POSTOPERATIVE STAGE

Immediately after the operation when the patient is able to co-operate, the régime of breathing exercises and simple leg movement is commenced. Treatment once daily is useless, and the patient must be encouraged to practise correct breathing at all times. Here the nurse is particularly helpful. In the early postoperative stages when the patient's co-operation is in doubt, the physiotherapist should attend for frequent short visits during the day.

Two sets of circumstances require additional measures:

1. Where the patient is failing to cough up accumulating secretions.

2. Where a blockage of a bronchial tube has occurred.

The additional measures required are postural drainage and/or chest shaking.

Postural drainage

This involves placing the patient in a position which allows gravity to assist in the removal of secretions from a lobe of the lung. The exact positioning used requires a detailed knowledge of the anatomy of the bronchial tree and information regarding the lobe or lobes of the lung affected. However, since the bases of the lungs are usually involved, modified positioning may be effective.

The end of the bed should be raised on blocks approximately 12 inches high.

The patient is then placed:

1. On the back with knees bent.
2. On the appropriate side with the knee bent.
3. On the face.

The presence of a drainage tube in the wound may complicate matters and it may be necessary to disconnect the tube temporarily. In some cases, it may not be possible to use position 3.

While in these positions the patient is encouraged to practise the breathing exercises, placing emphasis on a prolonged expiration. During expiration vigorous percussion or shaking is given by the physiotherapist to the chest wall and the patient encouraged to cough effectively.

Percussion and chest shaking

Percussion is given over the affected area by striking the chest wall repeatedly and alternately with lightly cupped hands, covering the part with a blanket which will reduce sting.

Shakings are given by grasping the front and back of the lower part of the rib cage between the outspread hands, and shaking vigorously. Avoid excessive pressure on the ribs.

THROMBUS FORMATION

If, in spite of physiotherapy, a thrombus does form, anti-coagulants are given immediately to try and prevent an embolus from appearing. Medical opinion is divided on whether or not leg and foot exercises should cease. It is probably safer to stop all exercise to the affected leg until the danger of embolus formation is past.

In postoperative physiotherapy prevention of complications is aimed at, and the success or failure of the methods outlined depends to a large extent on how successful is the physiotherapist in obtaining the co-operation of the patient.

Appendix 3

Tracheostomy regimen

PROCEDURE

The nurse must wear a mask as must *all visitors*.
1. Wash hands thoroughly before and after each manipulation.
2. Use catheters once only, then clean and replace in 'Hibitane' solution. Disposable catheters are to be preferred.
3. Use a catheter not more than half the diameter of the tracheostomy tube in thickness.
4. Touch only the proximal 3 inches of catheter with hands.
5. Do not let the catheter touch anything but the interior of the tube.
6. Use only gentle suction.
7. Manipulate the catheter gently in the trachea.
8. Enter both main bronchi by directing the tip of the catheter.
9. Flush the catheter with sterile water to clear it during use.
10. Unless otherwise instructed, only aspirate when necessary— i.e. if secretions can be heard bubbling in the air passages excessive use of the catheter can cause bleeding, spasm, increased secretions.
11. Aspirate only for a short period (e.g. 5 seconds) at any one time and allow adequate rest between periods.
12. The nurse will be instructed in the use of the humidifier and mucolytic or bronchodilating drugs if these are required.

13. Do not employ the same catheter for tracheal and nasal suction.

14. Care of tracheostomy tube and cuff: suck out pharynx first. The nurse will be instructed how often to deflate the cuff of the tracheostomy tube and how long the cuff has to remain deflated. The patient must never be fed orally or by stomach tube unless the cuff is inflated.

15. Vigorous physiotherapy is essential for these patients as is continual care of pressure points.

EQUIPMENT AT BEDSIDE (FIG. APPENDIX 3.1)

1. A spare sterile tracheostomy tube of the appropriate size in a sterile container.

2. Tape and scissors (sterile).

3. Gauze swabs (sterile).

4. Sterile lubricant

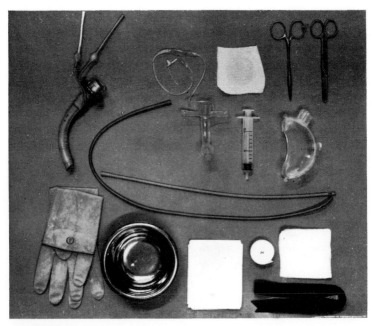

Figure Appendix 3.1 The tracheostomy tray.

5. Sterile tracheal suction catheters, preferably disposable or autoclaved and kept in a suitable dilution of Hibitane in a sterile container.

6. Tracheostomy box and supporting strap.

7. Sterile gloves

8. Sterile basin with sterile water or saline.

9. Artery forceps.

10. 10 ml syringe.

In addition, a bactericidal lotion for cleansing the area of the stoma should be available and 'Flexopad' rubber pads cut in such a way as to provide support for the tracheostomy tube.

Appendix 4

Scottish Home and Health Department: fires and explosion in operating theatres and anaesthetic rooms

WARNING NOTICE

Flammable anaesthetic agents such as ether, cyclopropane and ethyl chloride when mixed with air, oxygen or nitrous oxide may form explosive mixtures, and the ignition of such anaesthetic vapours has resulted in explosions which have been attended by serious consequences. The chief causes of such ignitions are:

1. Electrostatic spark discharge. This is more likely to occur during dry atmospheric conditions and in particular during the early part of a session when conditions tend to be driest.

2. Sparking at electrical contacts, diathermy electrodes etc.

3. Use of apparatus incorporating hot surfaces, e.g. cautery, electric heaters, overheated lamps.

4. Gas or spirit burners.

Whenever an explosive mixture is in use the surgeon and the theatre sister should be aware of the fact.

PRECAUTIONS AND RECOMMENDATIONS

1. Anti-static precautions

The best means of reducing electrostatic risks is to eliminate the use of materials which readily electrify in normal use. *The chief sources of static electricity are insulating rubber, plastics, wool, nylon.* Experience suggests that non-conducting rubber breathing equipment on anaesthetic apparatus constitutes the greater risk. Materials which are anti-static for practical purposes are available, e.g. anti-static rubber, anti-static rubber-proofed fabrics, linen, cotton and viscose, and should be used wherever possible instead of the electrostatic materials.

Recommended anti-static precautionary measures:

a. *Rubberised anaesthetic breathing equipment and rubber tubing* used with suction apparatus, etc. should have permanent anti-static properties.

b. *Operating tables, anaesthetic apparatus, patients' and other trolleys, stools, etc.,* should have metal or anti-static rubber-tyred castors or feet. The metal work of anaesthetic and other apparatus should be electrically continuous and top surfaces and shelves should be free from paint or other insulating finish.

c. *Rubber pads* on operating tables, trolleys or stools should have permanent anti-static properties or be completely enclosed in an anti-static fabric, e.g. cotton, linen or viscose rayon.

d. *All persons entering an anaesthetising location should wear anti-static footwear and a reasonably close-fitting outer garment of an anti-static fabric.* Anti-static rubber-soled footwear is considered preferable. Other types should be enclosed in overboots of an antistatic fabric, e.g. cotton or linen.

e. Floors should have suitable permanent anti-static properties, e.g. anti-static quality terrazzo, terrazzo tile, P.V.C. or ceramic tile floors.

2. Electrical apparatus

a. *Switch contacts* and other parts of apparatus capable of producing an incendive spark should be housed in a gas-tight enclosure or spaced at least 4 feet horizontally from any anaesthetic apparatus.

b. The maximum *voltage* of circuits used for energising endoscopes, etc., should be as *low* as is practicable and not appreciably higher than the rated voltage of the lamps. The provision of a special current limiting resistance in the circuit will greatly reduce the spark and overheating risks. *Dry-cell batteries* are safer than mains transformers for operating endoscopes.

c. *Electrically operated suction apparatus* should have no sparking contacts which are open to atmosphere, and the exhaust outlet from the pump should terminate outside any enclosure housing the apparatus.

d. From the electrical safety aspect *surgical tools* operated by means of compressed air are considered preferable to electrically-operated tools, because of the inherent spark and electric shock risks associated with the latter.

e. Flexible *cables* should be free from joints, frequently inspected and renewed when damaged or showing signs of deterioration.

f. The risks associated with *diathermy and cautery apparatus* are obvious. Before these are used following the administration of flammable anaesthetics a non-flammable gas should be passed through the breathing circuit until no explosive residue remains either in the apparatus or in the patient's lungs. The ether bottle and cyclopropane cylinder should be removed. It is not sufficient to rely on turning these taps off as they might not be gastight.

3. Open flames and heated surfaces

Apparatus incorporating open flame burners or heated surfaces which may operate at temperatures of 350°F (164°C) or more can constitute an ignition risk if located within 20 feet of an anaesthetising position. Doors between the anaesthetising position and the ignition risk should not be regarded as a reliable safeguard, as they may be left open.

Notes—Spirit lotions, etc. It should be noted that the use of spirit, spirit lotions and other flammable solutions which are frequently employed for cleansing the patient's skin, etc., involves dangers similar to those mentioned above. Additional information on the risks referred to above, together with recommended precautions against associated risks, are contained in 'Report of a Working Party on Anaesthetic Explosions' and Hospital Technical Memoranda Nos. 1 and 2 (H.M.S.O.).

FURTHER SAFETY PRECAUTIONS

In addition, there must be no smoking in the anaesthetic room or theatre precincts and *all theatre personnel* must be aware when an explosive mixture is in use. In any location where oxygen is being administered the precautions outlined in the warning notice should be observed. This applies equally to areas in general wards.

Appendix 5

Glasgow Royal Infirmary cardiac arrest chart

When external cardiac massage has been unsuccessful it is usual to proceed to the method of direct cardiac massage, following a thoracotomy. The urgency of this emergency is such that all present must know their individual tasks and carry them out quickly and efficiently. The necessary instruments and drugs, ready in packs, should be available in all operating theatres, recovery rooms and intensive care units. Apparatus such as electrical defibrillators and electrocardiograph machines must be kept available in some central position, known to all nursing and medical staff, to be sent for when required. It has been found of great assistance in many hospitals to outline the duties of all personnel on a wall chart. While this chart must be displayed in a convenient place it should not be in such a position that patients can see it.

Table Appendix 5.1 contains all the relevant information which is required to construct a wall chart. The Glasgow Royal Infirmary Cardiac Arrest Chart is based on this data but each hospital can, of course, decide upon the precise details of drugs, dosage, etc., and method of display, to suit local circumstances.

169

DON'T waste time. You have only 3 minutes to establish circulation.

DON'T give drugs until type and cause of arrest is determined.

DON'T wait for e.c.g. to begin treatment. An absent B.P. and absent pulse in a major vessel means cardiac arrest.

INITIAL EMERGENCY

1. Note the time.
2. Commence external cardiac massage immediately on firm surface.
3. Commence assistance to ventilation if necessary. (Mouth-to-Mouth breathing or bellows resuscitator.)
4. Send for resuscitation team and trolley. (Trolley carries e.c.g., defibrillator etc.)

DUTIES OF RESUSCITATION TEAM

(**Note:** In many cases the entire procedure can be followed without thoracotomy. Only if there is no response to the external methods is the chest opened).

ANAESTHETIST	SURGEON	ASSISTANT	NURSES
1. Establish a clear airway, e.g. endotracheal tube.	1. Continue external cardiac massage.	1. Connect e.c.g. leads to patient, confirm diagnosis, and observe e.c.g. constantly.	1. Assist anaesthetist with emergency syringes and transfusion equipment.
2. Ventilate lungs with 100% oxygen.	2. Apply external defibrillator electrodes if indicated.	2. Stand-by to relieve surgeon performing massage.	2. Keep note of time and events.
3. Tilt patient's head down 15 degrees.	3. If direct massage or internal defibrillation is indicated perform thoracotomy, i.e. open left 4th interspace transversely from sternal margin to mid-axillary line.	3. Operate defibrillation equipment if required.	3. Assist surgeon if thoracotomy is performed.
4. Check carotid pulse when cardiac massage is established.			
5. Check B.P.			
6. Set up intravenous infusion as vehicle for drugs.			

Table Appendix 5.1 Management of cardiac arrest.

POSSIBLE SITUATIONS EXISTING AFTER ADEQUATE MASSAGE AND OXYGENATION

1. THE HEART RESUMES A NORMAL BEAT	2. THE HEART REMAINS IN ARREST	
	(A) The heart is in fibrillation	(B) The heart is in asystole
(a) Continue massage in rhythm with beat until the B.P. is maintained at a minimum of 80 mm Hg systolic.	(a) Carry out electrical defibrillation external or internal and continue adequate massage between shocks.	(a) Continue adequate massage.
(b) If contractions do not improve give adrenaline 1:1000, 0.5–1 ml (diluted to 10 ml with sterile water) into the cavity of the right ventricle.	(b) Administer 0.8% sodium bicarbonate intravenously to correct acidosis (100 mmol for average adult).	(b) Give calcium chloride 10%, 5–10 ml, intravenously or into the cavity of the right ventricle.
(c) If contractions are fairly good but B.P. remains low give in 500 ml 5% glucose, slowly intravenously.	(c) If spontaneous beat returns follow column 1.	(c) Give 0.8% sodium bicarbonate intravenously to correct acidosis (100 mmol for average adult).
(d) In all cases give sodium bicarbonate intravenously to correct acidosis (100 mmol for the average adult).	(d) If heart is in asystole follow column 2B.	(d) If asystole persists give adrenaline 1:1000, 0.5–1 ml (diluted to 10 ml with sterile water) into cavity of right ventricle.
(e) If thoracotomy has been performed close chest with adequate haemostasis and water-seal drain.		(e) If heart beat returns follow column 1.
		(f) If asystole persists continue massage up to 1 hour or until heart fails to fill in diastole.

Table Appendix 5.1 (*continued*)

Glossary

Amnesia
A state of forgetfulness. Usually this is a valuable property of premedicant drugs as unpleasant episodes are forgotten postoperatively.

Analgesia
Freedom from pain; it must be distinguished from **anaesthesia**, which means absence of all sensation.

Ataractic drugs
Those which produce a state of indifference in the patient to his surroundings.

Atelectasis
A state in which lung alveoli are collapsed and airless, taking no part in respiration.

Autonomic nervous system
'Independent' nervous system; used to describe the sympathetic and parasympathetic nervous systems. This is in contrast to the **somatic** nerves, which carry painful sensation to the brain and motor impulses from the brain to the different parts of the body.

Bradycardia
An excessive slowing of the heart rate.

Bronchodilator drugs Those which relax the smooth muscle surrounding the bronchi.

Cardiac catheterisation A diagnostic technique used mainly in patients with congenital heart disease. A catheter is passed by way of a vein into the various parts of the heart and great vessels.

Controlled ventilation A term used to describe the inflation of the lungs by the anaesthetist, after the patient's own respiratory efforts have been abolished. The technique is commonly termed intermittent positive pressure ventilation (IPPV) and may be carried out manually or by a mechanical ventilator.

Dead space air The volume of air which fills the nose, mouth and bronchi during each inspiration. Since it never reaches the alveoli it does not play any part in respiration.

Eclampsia A complication of pregnancy characterised by high blood pressure, albuminuria and convulsions.

Emetics Drugs which induce vomiting.

Euphoria A feeling of well-being characteristically associated with morphine and allied drugs.

Elective operations Those which can be performed at a time chosen to suit the parties concerned. They contrast with **emergency** procedures where the operation is performed as soon as possible to save life.

Endoscopy A term used to describe bronchoscopy and oesophagoscopy, cystoscopy and other similar investigations. Literally it means 'looking into'.

Hypothermia

Used to describe a state where the body temperature is lower than normal. This state is often intentionally induced. **Hyperthermia**, on the other hand, where the temperature is unduly raised, is usually associated with pathological conditions, e.g. head injuries, toxic effects of drugs.

Hypoxaemia

A state where the blood carries less than the normal amount of oxygen to the tissues. This is often incorrectly called **anoxaemia**, which means the absence of oxygen. Quite severe hypoxaemia may exist without **cyanosis**.

Intensive care units

Intended to care for selected patients requiring concentrated medical and nursing attention. The patients may be in such a unit for a period varying from days to weeks. **The recovery room** is, in contrast, intended to deal with most or all patients in the immediate postoperative period and the patients will normally leave this room after a maximum period of 24 hours.

Mucolytics

Drugs used to liquefy mucus.

Narcotics

Agents which produce drowsiness, sleep, stupor or insensibility. A volatile narcotic is one which can be given as a gas or vapour in contrast to injections such as morphine (non-volatile narcotics).

Paraplegia

A state in which the lower limbs and part or all of the trunk are paralysed.

Peripheral circulation

Circulation to the more distant parts of the body. In this work, usually used to describe the blood flow through the skin, subcutaneous tissues and muscle.

Sedatives

Drugs which soothe a patient.

Sensory cortex The part of the brain where impulses from the organs are appreciated as pain, etc. The **motor cortex** is the part of the brain which sends out impulses which cause movements to take place.

Side-effects (of drugs) Those which occur in addition to the main effect for which the drug is given. Thus when morphine is given to relieve pain (main effect) it may produce euphoria (desirable side-effect) and vomiting (undesirable side-effect).

Soda-lime Used in some anaesthetic machines to absorb carbon dioxide from the patient's exhalations.

Specific muscle relaxants Those which cause muscles to relax without producing other effects on the body. Curare is such a drug. Ether and other potent anaesthetic agents, which produce unconsciousness and other effects in addition to muscular relaxation, are known as non-specific relaxants.

Toxic effects Those which occur when excessive doses of a drug are given.

Tracheostomy The term used to describe the formation of an opening in the trachea through the neck, often to enable a tube to be inserted. **Tracheotomy** merely describes the cutting into the trachea.

Further reading

Campbell D, Spence A A 1978 Norris & Campbell's Anaesthetics, resuscitation and intensive care, 5th edn. Churchill Livingstone, Edinburgh

Moir D D 1982 Pain relief in labour, 4th edn. Churchill Livingstone, Edinburgh

Index